Eating Behaviors of the Young Child
Prenatal and Postnatal Influences on Healthy Eating

Edited by
Leann Birch, PhD
William Dietz, MD, PhD

American Academy of Pediatrics
141 Northwest Point Blvd
Elk Grove Village, IL 60007-1098

Supported by an educational grant from the Johnson & Johnson Pediatric Institute, L.L.C.

The Johnson & Johnson Pediatric Institute, L.L.C. (JJPI), is dedicated to advancing maternal and children's health worldwide. By working in partnership with leading healthcare professionals and organizations, JJPI creates educational initiatives to improve the lives of children and their families, and build on the Johnson & Johnson heritage of caring for mothers and babies.

The AAP and JJPI gratefully acknowledge Karin Gillespie, MBA, for her dedicated efforts as technical editor of this publication. Her valued input, persistence and devotion are greatly appreciated.

Table of Contents

Table of Contents (continued)

Participants

Peggy Bentley, PhD
Professor of Nutrition
Associate Dean for Global Health
School of Public Health
University of North Carolina at Chapel Hill
CB# 7461
4115C McGavran-Greenberg
Chapel Hill, North Carolina 27599 USA

Leann Birch, PhD
Distinguished Professor of Human Development
Department of Human Development/Family Studies
Pennsylvania State University
College of Health and Human Development
129 Noll Laboratory
University Park, Pennsylvania 16802 USA

Christina J. Calamaro PhD, CRNP
Post Doctoral Fellow
Center for Sleep and Respiratory Neurobiology
University of Pennsylvania Schools of Medicine and Nursing
420 Guardian Drive
Philadelphia, Pennsylvania 19104 USA

Tim Cole, BA, B.Phil, MA, PhD, ScD
Professor of Medical Statistics
Paediatric Epidemiology and Biostatistics Unit
Institute of Child Health
University College of London
30 Guilford Street
London, England, WC1N 1EH

Barbara Devaney, PhD
Vice President
Mathematica Policy Research
P.O. Box 2393
Princeton, New Jersey 08543 USA

Kathryn Dewey, PhD
Professor
Department of Nutrition
University of California Davis Medical Center
3253A Meyer Hall
One Shields Avenue
Davis, California 95616 USA

William Dietz, MD, PhD
Director of Nutrition and Physical Activity
Centers for Disease Control and Prevention
1600 Clifton Road
Atlanta, Georgia 30333 USA

Richard Fiene, PhD
Associate Professor
Human Development and Family Studies
Pennsylvania State University–Harrisburg
W-311B Olmstead Building
777 West Harrisburg Pike
Middletown, Pennsylvania 17057 USA

Jennifer Orlet Fisher, PhD
Assistant Professor
Department of Pediatrics
Baylor College of Medicine
One Baylor Plaza
Mail Stop BCM320
Houston, Texas 77030 USA

Sir David M. B. Hall, MB, BS, BSc, FRCPCH, FRCP, FFPHM (Hon.), FRCP (Edin.)
Professor of Community Paediatrics
University of Sheffield and the University of the NHS
Honorary Consultant Paediatrician
Sheffield Children's Trust
Storrs House Farm
Storrs Lane Stannington
Sheffield, England, S6 6GY

Participants (continued)

Robert C. Hornik, PhD
Wilbur Schramm Professor of Communication
Annenberg School of Communication
University of Pennsylvania
3620 Walnut Street
Philadelphia, Pennsylvania 19104 USA

Jon Korfmacher, PhD
Associate Professor
Erikson Institute
420 North Wabash Avenue
6th Floor
Chicago, Illinois 60611 USA

Donna Matheson, PhD
Senior Research Scientist
Stanford Prevention Research Center
Stanford University School of Medicine
211 Quarry Drive, Room N229
Hoover Pavilion, Mail Code 5705
Stanford, California 94305 USA

David Mechlin, MBA
Senior Partner
Worldwide Client Service Director
Ogilvy & Mather
309 West 49th Street
New York, New York 10019 USA

Julie Mennella, PhD
Researcher
Monell Chemical Senses Center
3500 Market Street
Philadelphia, Pennsylvania 19104 USA

Kenneth Resnicow, PhD
Professor
Health Behavior & Health Education
School of Public Health
University of Michigan
M5009 SPII
109 Observatory Street
Ann Arbor, Michigan 48109 USA

Thomas Robinson, MD, MPH
Associate Professor of Pediatrics and Medicine
Division of General Pediatrics & Stanford Prevention Research Center
Director, Center for Healthy Weight
Lucile Packard Children's Hospital at Stanford
Stanford University School of Medicine
Hoover Pavilion, Room N229
211 Quarry Drive, Mail Code 5705
Stanford, California 94305 USA

Mary Rudolf, MB, BS, BSc, DCH, MRCPCH, FAAP
Professor
Consultant Paediatrician
University of Leeds
Belmont House
3-5 Belmont Grove
Leeds, England, LS2 9DE

Bettylou Sherry, PhD
Epidemiologist
Maternal and Child Nutrition Branch
Division of Nutrition and Physical Activity
Centers for Disease Control and Prevention
NCCDPHP/DNPA/MCN, Mail Stop K-25
4700 Buford Highway, NE
Atlanta, Georgia 30341 USA

Elizabeth Vandewater, PhD
Associate Professor
Human Development and Family Sciences
University of Texas at Austin
1 University Station
Austin, Texas 78712 USA

Preface

Feeding an infant or toddler a varied, healthful diet is one of the most important — and often most challenging — tasks of early parenting. The eating behaviors children learn and adopt in infancy and as toddlers affect their nutrition and health in childhood, adolescence and even into adulthood. Good feeding involves a reciprocal relationship — in a sense, a dance between child and parent. The research tells us that most parents and children learn this dance well — and their children transition smoothly from breast and bottle feeding to solid foods and a sound family diet. But an increasing number of parents and children falter — and their children make poor food choices, eat beyond satiety and fill up on sweet drinks rather than healthy solids.

A multidisciplinary faculty convened a Pediatric Round Table supported by an educational grant from the Johnson & Johnson Pediatric Institute, L.L.C. to explore this most pressing public health issue of young children and feeding. The faculty participants included pediatricians, researchers, policymakers, social scientists, anthropologists, communications professionals and academicians recognized globally for their work in child health, feeding, nutrition and growth. The culmination of the Pediatric Round Table — beyond the lively discussion, dialogue and debate that occur during the meeting— is the development over 18 months and publication of this educational book for health care providers and other child health professionals.

The overall objectives for the Pediatric Round Table were ambitious:

- To review current knowledge about how to promote the development of healthy eating behaviors during the first 5 years of life
- To use state-of-the-art communication models and methods to develop a plan for disseminating a public health message and guidance to promote healthy eating from birth (and even before birth) to 5 years

Selecting and effectively communicating a set of evidence-based messages, for healthcare and child care professionals, and ultimately for parents, was the goal of the Pediatric Round Table.

A number of themes emerged from the discussion:

- An emphasis on good nutrition and a varied diet for infants and young children should begin even before birth
- Mothers who breastfeed expose their infants to a wealth of flavor experiences that prime them to more readily accept novel foods as toddlers and young children. Children who are fed formula are not exposed to these varied flavor experiences
- Mother's milk and amniotic fluid reflect her culture. Food habits are perhaps the most enduring aspect of a culture, and through her diet during pregnancy and breastfeeding, a mother transmits the flavors of her culture to her child
- Parents can learn how to practice responsive feeding, guided by a child's cues and satiety signals
- Children are eating and feeding today in a new environment of plenty. High calorie, high fat food is available wherever they go — and often children are eating in settings away from home and parents. Evolution did not prepare us for this overabundance
- Effective public health interventions are needed now — even before we have all the answers on the factors driving the increase in overweight and obesity. It's better to intervene and examine the results than it is to simply observe the status quo. Interventions are needed all along the life span

These themes and others — which emphasize the critical role that parents and healthcare providers play in helping children develop healthy eating habits — are explored in detail in the chapters that follow.

Introduction

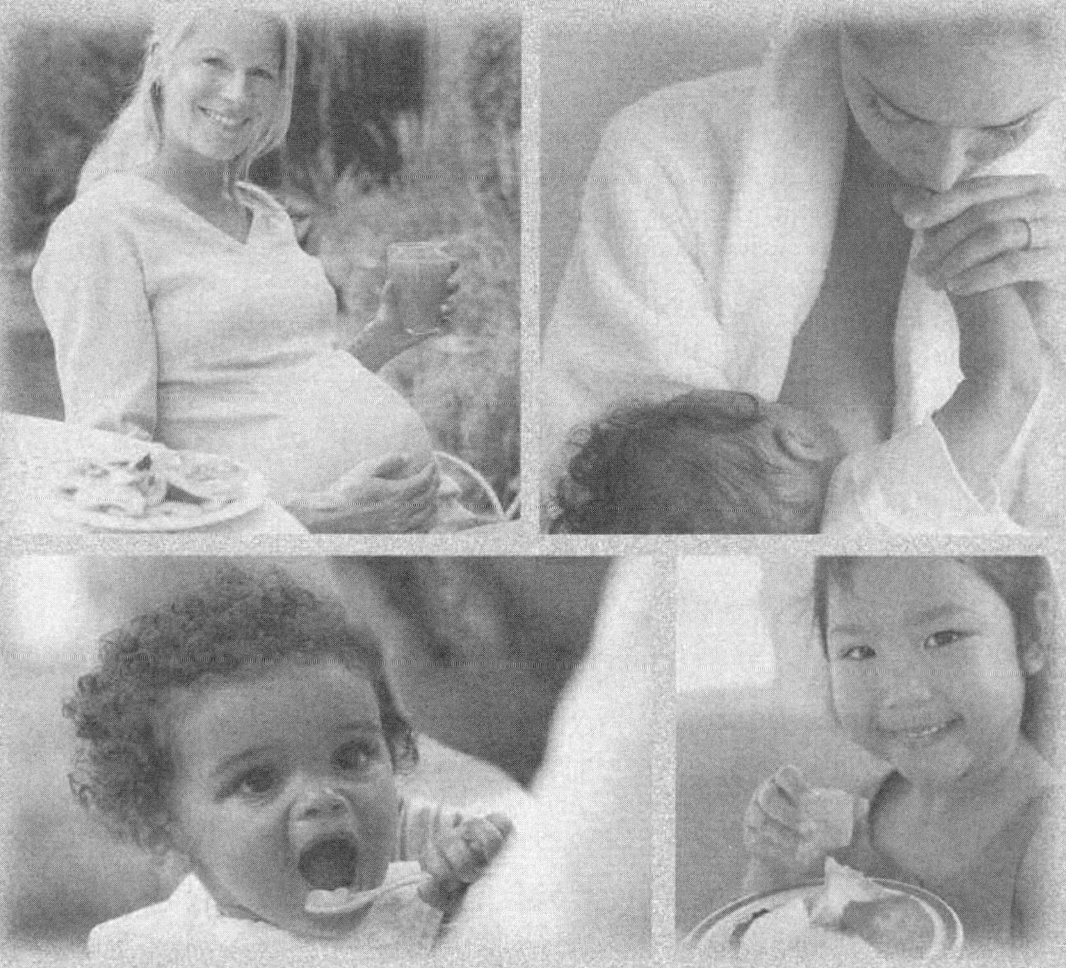

Introduction

Leann Birch, PhD

Young Children and Eating: What Do We Know and What Do We Need to Do?

The first 5 years of life are a period of rapid growth and change, when adequate nutrition is critical to healthy development. One of the challenges for healthcare professionals is to clearly describe and define growth patterns during this early period, and to provide guidelines and tools to distinguish children who are growing well — within normal limits — from those children who fall below or exceed those norms. The chapter by Donna Matheson, PhD, and Thomas Robinson, MD, MPH, and another chapter by Tim Cole, PhD, ScD, in this book address the definition of childhood obesity and its comorbidities.

Breast Versus Bottle

We now know that the first feeding choice that parents make, whether to breastfeed or formula feed their baby, shapes individual differences in growth and metabolism, and influences infants' subsequent food preferences and eating patterns. (For more information, see the chapters in this volume by Julie Mennella, PhD, and Kathryn Dewey, PhD.) Because the flavor of human milk changes as a function of the mother's dietary intake, the breastfed infant experiences and becomes familiar with a variety of flavors from the adult diet of their culture, providing a "flavor bridge" that can promote the acceptance of solid foods later on. In contrast, the formula-fed infant does not have the opportunity to experience flavors from the adult diet, and the flavor experience is limited to that provided by the formula. In addition to the differences in early flavor experiences of formula-fed and breastfed infants, there are differences in how active a role the infant plays in determining intake. The breastfed infant plays a much more active role in determining the pace of the feeding and the volume of milk consumed at each feeding than does the formula-fed infant. Differences in dyadic interactions during breast and formula feeding may also lead subsequently to differences in maternal feeding practices and in the child's regulation of energy intake. Characterization of differences in early feeding styles can reveal how eating behavior is shaped by the parent-child interactions that occur around feeding and, in particular, how specific feeding styles may place children at risk for the development of eating problems and failure to thrive. The chapter by Professor Mary Rudolf discusses this in more detail.

Breastfeeding has a modest protective effect against childhood obesity, and it is widely recognized that the growth patterns of breastfed and formula-fed infants differ. (See the chapter in this volume by Kathryn Dewey, PhD.) The new growth norms of the World Health Organization (see www.who.int/childgrowth/en/index.html) reflect these differences. Rates of breastfeeding initiation have increased dramatically in recent years, and current rates of initiation are approaching the goal of Healthy People 2010, which is an initiation rate of 75% in the United States. However, progress in increasing the duration and exclusivity of breastfeeding has been slow, and the prevalence of breastfeeding among low-income and minority groups remains well below the national average.[1] Increasing the duration and exclusivity of breastfeeding by minority groups, who are at high risk for poor nutrition and childhood obesity, is a top priority. One promising approach to promoting breastfeeding among low-income minority mothers is described in the chapter by Jon Korfmacher, PhD, in this volume. In addition, research by Peggy Bentley, PhD, (who presented a video at the Round Table) and her colleagues[2] on infant feeding practices among low-income black mothers provides insight into the barriers to breastfeeding, and the prevalence of early introduction of solid foods, and can inform the design of interventions to promote healthier feeding patterns.

The Transition to Table Food

During the early years of life, a dramatic dietary change occurs as infants transition from a diet consisting exclusively of breast milk or formula to a diet that is very similar to that eaten by the adults around him or her. (See the chapter by Barbara Devaney, PhD, and Mary Kay Fox, MEd, for further discussion.) This begins a period of autonomy in feeding: The diet is initially "parent-selected" but becomes increasingly "child-selected." This evolution is accelerated in those environments where the time allotted to food preparation is no longer the limiting factor in the food that is available to the child. In current eating environments, parents have a range of choices among palatable, inexpensive, ready-to-eat foods that require little or no preparation. However, healthy food choices are often limited, few fruits and vegetables are offered, and many of the foods that are offered are palatable because they are high in energy density, fat, sugar and salt. One unintended consequence of these new food environments is that setting limits on food choices has become increasingly challenging for parents, who may allow even very young children the autonomy to choose and eat preferred foods, potentially compromising diet quality.

Because children's food preferences play a central role in shaping their dietary intake, it is especially critical that we take steps to help toddlers and young children learn to prefer nutritious foods by making these foods attractive and readily available, and having the adults around them serve as positive role models for healthy eating. How do current eating environments influence young children's dietary intake? Aspects of this broad question are addressed by several chapters in this volume, including those by Julie Mennella, PhD; Kathryn Dewey, PhD; Jennifer Orlet Fisher, PhD, and Leann Birch, PhD; Barbara Devaney, PhD and Mary Kay Fox, MEd; and Elizabeth Vandewater, PhD. We do know that eating environments play a powerful role in shaping patterns of intake. As young omnivores, children are predisposed to accept the foods available in their environments, but they also enter the world with a predisposition toward basic sweet and salty tastes.

Children, therefore, have to learn to like complex food flavors, and this learning occurs through their early eating experiences. Children acquire food preferences as they associate food cues with the social contexts and physiological consequences of eating.[3] As parents, caregivers and other adults introduce young children to new foods, children learn to like and eat these foods when they have repeated positive experiences with them. Modeling — giving children opportunities to see other children and adults consuming healthy foods — can also foster preferences for and willingness to eat new foods.[4]

Food Preferences Among Young Children

What kinds of foods are young children regularly eating today? Barbara Devaney, PhD and Mary Kay Fox, MEd, address this question in their study of infants and toddlers, using a nationally representative sample. Their data clearly illustrate the dramatic dietary transition that occurs between 6 and 24 months of age — as the diet shifts from predominately milk or formula (with about 80% of energy provided by milk or formula) to predominately table food (with about 80% of energy provided by table foods and sweetened drinks).

Therefore, the period from 6 to 24 months of age provides perhaps our best opportunity to shape healthier eating habits. If families consume green and yellow vegetables rather than French fries, the youngest members of the family will learn to eat vegetables. Before the first birthday, an infant is well on the way to transitioning from eating weanling foods to eating the very same "table foods" that are consumed by other family members. The data from Devaney and Fox (in this volume) reveal that at around 1 year of age, diet quality may be "as good as it gets." In fact, the indicators show that diet quality begins to decline around that time.

Other research indicates that declines in the quality of children's diets continue throughout childhood and adolescence, and into young adulthood.[5] The observed declines begin with the introduction of table foods from the adult diet; French fries rapidly become the most commonly consumed vegetable, taking the place of green and yellow vegetables.

Cultural Influences on Children's Food Preferences

Infants learn to accept and eat foods they are offered by other members of their culture. As such, in today's eating environments, they learn to accept — and actually prefer — many of the dietary choices that contribute to the epidemic of overweight and obesity among children and adults. The simple answer to the question, "How can we promote healthy eating habits among our children from birth to 5 years of age?" is the following: "By promoting healthier food choices among their parents." This is a tall order. As the 2005 Institute of Medicine report, *Preventing Childhood Obesity: Health in the Balance,*[6] makes clear, to support parents and children in making healthier food choices and adopting healthier activity patterns will require changes in the broad range of economic, social and environmental factors that shape the marketplace and provide the context for choice. For parents, food choices for themselves and their children involve trade-offs among taste, cost, convenience and health consequences. Recent evidence reveals that parents' child feeding practices and children's intake patterns differ across income and ethnic groups. In the chapter by Barbara Devaney, PhD, and Mary Kay Fox, MEd, dietary intake patterns of infants and toddlers are described. When the findings are stratified by income and ethnicity, children from low-income and minority families are more likely to eat foods high in calories but low in other essential nutrients. In the chapter by Bettylou Sherry, PhD, RD, and colleagues, we see that parental concerns about feeding their children, as well as the child feeding practices they use, also differ across income and ethnicity. (See the chapter by Fisher and Birch in this volume.) Taken together, these findings make it clear that interventions will need to be tailored to ethnicity and income; "one size fits all" interventions are unlikely to succeed.

Changes in Eating Environments

Our eating environments have changed dramatically in recent decades. Shifts in economic and social factors have altered the family structure, childcare practices and settings, food availability and preparation, and children's eating environments in general. With more mothers of young children working outside the home, an increasing number of children are cared for away from home — and they are consuming foods prepared and served there. Currently, nearly half of the family food budget is spent on "food away from home," which includes foods prepared and/or eaten away from home. Family meals — which typically provide more nutritious foods for children[7] as well as a context for socialization about food and eating — are on the decline because of time constraints and conflicting family member schedules.[8] In addition, limited descriptive data indicate that children's meals often are served in front of the TV.[9] However, at this point, we know relatively little about how young children's eating is influenced by concomitant TV viewing. In her chapter, Elizabeth Vandewater, PhD, discusses the link between television viewing and childhood obesity.

Intervening to Prevent Obesity and Shape Healthy Diets

In addition to concerns about the declining quality of young children's diets, there are concerns about the growing problem of overweight among young children: 26% of children 2 to 5 years of age are at risk of becoming overweight.[10] This startling statistic underscores the urgency of identifying efficacious approaches to promote healthy eating behaviors. To date, most obesity-prevention programs have focused on older children (whose food preferences and eating habits are already shaped), and only a few of these programs have had much success.[11]

The evidence presented in this volume provides us with key findings that can inform the design of new intervention approaches. Given that it is easier to establish new habits than to alter existing ones and that early dietary intake patterns can have an impact on later ones, a focus on this early period as the time to foster healthy eating habits makes sense. In fact, the findings suggest that early interventions may be more successful than those targeted at school-aged children and adolescents.

The research reviewed in this volume suggests a number of promising intervention strategies.

- Healthcare professionals, policymakers, parents and childcare professionals can help foster children's preferences for healthy foods — especially fruits and vegetables and complex carbohydrates — by promoting early flavor experiences via breastfeeding and encouraging the availability of healthy foods in home and daycare settings.
- Healthcare professionals can provide parents with information on setting limits for food quantities and offering healthy food choices.
- With information provided by healthcare professionals and childcare providers, parents can learn how to set eating limits for their children, offer and promote eating of healthy foods, and support the development of self-regulation of food intake by their children.
- With guidance on monitoring children's eating and responsive parenting, parents can learn to identify hunger in their children, discriminate it from other distress cues and recognize satiety signals. By understanding hunger and satiety, parents can offer food only in response to hunger and use alternative techniques for reducing other distress.

These interventions have the potential to reduce overfeeding and excessive weight gain, but are yet untested.

Although the data are limited and many important questions are still unanswered, the collected work in this volume reveals that the first 5 years of life offer enormous opportunities to promote healthier patterns of food intake.

These first years are a critical time period for transmission of cultural and familial attitudes, beliefs and practices about food and eating; development of food preferences; regulation of energy intake and energy balance; and prevention of overweight and obesity. In addition, the data on tracking of food and nutrient intake during development suggest that interventions that positively impact very early patterns of food intake may continue to have a positive impact on patterns of intake later on. So far, few systematic attempts have been made to intervene and promote healthier patterns of intake among our youngest children. The evidence presented by Devaney and colleagues in this volume and elsewhere[12] suggest that many of the problems apparent in the diets of older children could have emerged during the first years of life, underscoring the need for such early interventions.

Effective interventions that support parents, healthcare professionals and daycare providers (see the chapter by Richard Fiene, PhD) have taken on new urgency in light of the evidence, albeit limited, that declines in diet quality begin during the first year of life, as well as the continued increases in the prevalence of childhood overweight affecting children as early as birth to 5 years of age.

The material discussed in the chapters that follow represents the most recent advances in our knowledge of the factors that influence early eating patterns. Ultimately, the goal is to use this information to develop educational materials for parents and caregivers that will promote healthy eating in young children. Our hope is that by extracting key messages from the new knowledge presented here, in combination with what is known about producing positive changes in health behaviors, we can develop a set of teaching and learning materials that support parents and caregivers in their efforts to help children develop healthier eating behaviors during the early years of life.

References

1. Ryan AS, Zhou W. Lower breastfeeding rates persist among the special supplemental nutrition program for women, infants, and children participants, 1978-2003. *Pediatrics.* 2006;117:1136-1146.
2. Bronner YL, Gross SM, Caulfield L, et al. Early introduction of solid foods among urban African-American participants in WIC. *Journal of the American Dietetic Association.* 99;4:457-461.
3. Birch LL. Development of food preferences. Annual Review of Nutrition. 1999;19:41-62.
4. Fisher JO, Mitchell DC, Smiciklas-Wright H, Mannino ML, Birch LL. Meeting calcium recommendations during middle childhood reflects mother-daughter beverage choices and predicts bone mineral status. *American Journal of Clinical Nutrition.* 2004;79:698-706.

5. Mannino ML, Lee Y, Mitchell DC, Smiciklas-Wright H, Birch LL. The quality of girls' diets declines and tracks across middle childhood. *International Journal of Behavioral Nutrition and Physical Activity.* 2004;1(5):1-11.
6. Koplan JP, Liverman CT, Kraak VI, eds. *Preventing Childhood Obesity: Health in the Balance.* Washington, DC: National Academy Press; 2005.
7. Patrick H, Nicklas TA. A review of family and social determinants of children's eating patterns and diet quality. *Journal of the American College of Nutrition.* 2005;2:83-92.
8. Larson R, Wiley A, Branscomb K. *Family Meals as Contexts of Development and Socialization.* New Directions for Child and Adolescent Development, No. 111. San Francisco, Ca: Jossey-Bass; 2006.
9. Sherry B, McDivitt J, Birch LL, et al. Attitudes, practices, and concerns about child feeding and child weight status among socioeconomically diverse Caucasian, Hispanic and African-American mothers. *Journal of the American Dietetic Association.* 2004;104:215-221.
10. Ogden CL, Carroll MD, Curtin LR, McDowell MA, Tabak CJ, Flegal KM. Prevalence of overweight and obesity in the United States. *Journal of the American Medical Association.* 2006;295:1549-1555.
11. Jeffery RW, Linde JA. Evolving environmental factors in the obesity epidemic. In: Crawford D, Jeffery RW, eds. *Obesity Prevention and Public Health.* Oxford England: Oxford University Press; 2005.
12. Fox MK, Reidy K, Karwe V, Ziegler P. Average portions of foods commonly eaten by infants and toddlers in the United States. *Journal of the American Dietetic Association.* 2006;106:s66-s76.

Section 1
Nutrition Influences on Growth and Development

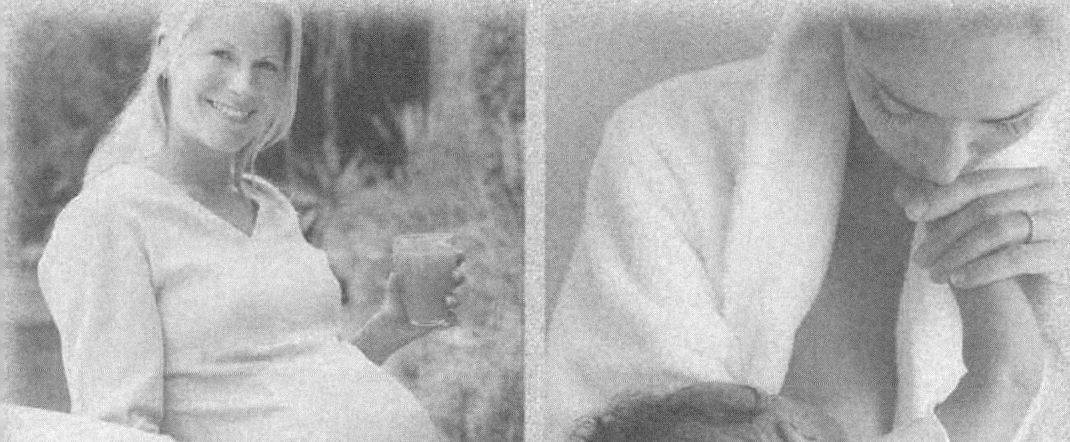

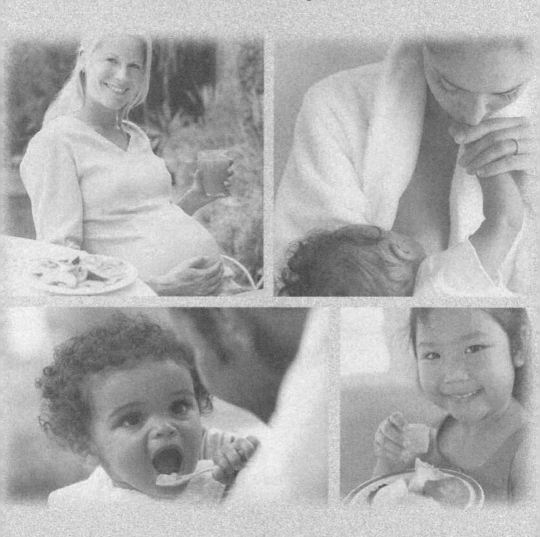

Abstracts From Section 1 Nutrition Influences on Growth and Development

Measuring Normal Growth and Growth Variance in Infancy and Childhood

Tim J. Cole, ScD

Pediatrics is the medical specialty that focuses on the care and treatment of children from birth through their late teens. A fundamental part of pediatrics is monitoring the growth and development of infants and children. Although growth charts for weight and height are important guidelines during infancy and childhood, they are poor indicators of growth velocity. Thrive lines lend a useful additional perspective. Thrive lines are a set of lines, available on a transparent plastic overlay, that are placed on top of the weight chart and indicate the amount of centile crossing corresponding to the 5th weight velocity centile over a 4-week period. Healthcare providers now know that height adjustment based on family history improves the accuracy of height assessment, and body mass index (BMI) is better proxy for adiposity than is weight. Although childhood height is an effective predictor for adult height, BMI varies from child to adult. Both low birth weight and high postnatal weight gain predict a later adverse outcome (eg, obesity, insulin resistance or hypertension). One researcher's "growth acceleration" hypothesis proposes that rapid weight gain is a causal risk factor for obesity. The link between weight gain, diet and health outcomes may, in fact, be driven by appetite, which suggests that there is a role for the newly discovered hormone ghrelin.

Obesity in Young Children

Donna M. Matheson, PhD
Thomas N. Robinson, MD, MPH

Obesity — which is correlated positively with morbidity, mortality, and social and economic costs — has increased rapidly among both children and adults in the United States and other countries. Childhood obesity, in particular, is a significant public health problem. Compared to what is known about the causes, correlations and consequences of obesity in older children, adolescents and adults, very little is known about obesity in young children. Body mass index (BMI) appears to be the most practical and appropriate measure to define overweight in young children. Young children are generally considered obese if their body mass index (BMI, kg/m^2) is at or above the 95th percentile of a particular reference (eg, the 2000 Centers for Disease Control and Prevention BMI references or the International Obesity Taskforce BMI references). Although data are sparse, BMI in young children modestly predicts later adult obesity, and is associated with increased cardiovascular disease risk factors. It is not yet clear whether BMI in early childhood predicts adult morbidity and mortality. Despite gaps in our knowledge, however, there appears to be adequate support for interventions in childhood to prevent and control overweight. There is a critical need for more experimental research to develop effective and practical interventions for parents and families, caregivers, educators, health professionals, institutions and policymakers.

Prenatal and Postnatal Flavor Learning in Human Infants

Julie A. Mennella, PhD

A fundamental feature of mammals is that their first foods — amniotic fluid and mother's milk — are flavored by the foods eaten by the mother during pregnancy and lactation, respectively. These first taste experiences bias infants' acceptance of particular flavors and may "program" their later food preferences. Infants' acceptance of a flavor may not require that they experience that particular flavor in utero or during lactation. However, experience with a variety of flavors in utero and during lactation increases the likelihood that infants will accept a variety of novel foods during weaning.

Breastfeeding and Other Infant Feeding Practices That May Influence Child Obesity

Kathryn G. Dewey, PhD

New studies on the relationship between breastfeeding and child obesity have sparked interest in this issue, especially in light of the continuing trend towards higher rates of child obesity in the United States and other countries. This chapter examines findings on weight differences between breastfed and formula-fed infants in infancy, childhood and adolescence; offers some explanations for the association between breastfeeding and the lower risk of child overweight; and looks at other common feeding practices that may influence obesity. The author subsequently discusses the clinical and public health implications of child obesity and offers some promising intervention strategies.

Measuring Normal Growth and Growth Variance in Infancy and Childhood

Tim J. Cole, ScD

Introduction

Any discussion of feeding practices in infancy and early childhood should take into consideration the growth of the child. At the simplest level, a child who grows rapidly tends to eat more than does a child who grows more slowly.[1] The correlation between dietary intake and growth is driven by the child's appetite: A hungry child eats more and tends to grow faster.[2,3] (The composition of the child's diet also influences the child's body composition later in life.[4]) The obvious question of which came first — appetite driving growth or growth driving appetite — is a chicken-and-egg question that is currently unanswerable. However, without a doubt, the diet-appetite-growth triad is a critical issue in infant and child feeding.

As Professor John Davis has memorably said, "Pediatrics is the medicine of growth and development."[2] Monitoring growth is a fundamental part of medical assessment in infancy and childhood because normal growth is a proxy for health. When children are healthy, they typically grow well. Conversely, when children are ill, even if they do not have an explicit growth disorder, their growth is likely to be negatively affected, too. The very importance of growth assessment, thus, makes the routine use of growth charts an essential part of pediatric practice. The first part of this chapter describes how growth charts should be used, with a particular focus on children's weight and height.

Growth in infancy and early childhood is an indicator of current health, as well as a harbinger of adult size and health. An individual's size and health in late childhood, adolescence and adulthood can be predicted to some degree by size and growth patterns during early life. These 2 correlations — of early growth with later size and early growth with later health outcomes — also are discussed separately in this chapter.

Measurement of Growth

Growth Reference Charts

The neonate's first anthropometry measurement is birth weight. Subsequent weight measurements provide a simple and effective summary of an infant's growth pattern. At any particular age, an infant's weight is a measure of "weight distance" in Tanner's terminology, while the rate of change in weight over time is a measure of "weight velocity."[3] Traditionally, weight charts measure weight distance, which is expressed as a centile or z score relative to a reference population. The weight centile indicates the percentage of the reference population of the same age and sex that weighs less than the child does (eg, for a child in the 75th centile, 75% of the reference population weighs less). The z score represents the number of standard deviations (SDs) that the child's weight is above or below the median for his or her age and sex. There is a direct link between centile and z score via the normal distribution, so that the 75th centile corresponds to 0.67 SDs above the median.[4]

Many countries have developed their own weight charts, for example the British 1990 weight chart (British 1990),[5] the United States Centers for Disease Control and Prevention 2000 growth chart (US CDC 2000)[6] and the Dutch 1997 growth chart (Dutch 1997).[7] Because the distribution of weight is skewed at most ages, these charts are constructed using the LMS method, which adjusts for this skewness.[8] The reference data are largely cross-sectional, with each child contributing a single measurement. Therefore, the charts contain no information on growth velocity. When using the charts, it is assumed that a child growing "normally" stays on the same centile over time, a pattern called tracking. Conversely, when children grow faster or slower than average, their weight centile changes over time, a pattern known as centile crossing.

Figure 1 is the male infant weight chart from the British 1990 reference.[5] The chart consists of 9 centile curves, each spaced two thirds of an SD apart, with the 0.4th and 99.6th centiles at the lower and upper ends of the continuum, respectively. These centiles were selected as endpoints to minimize the false-positive screening rate.[9] The weight chart shows a growth curve for a hypothetical child, which I discuss in the next section.

Figure 1. The British 1990 boys weight chart from birth to 12 months of age, with a hypothetical child weighed at 7, 8 and 9 months of age.[5]

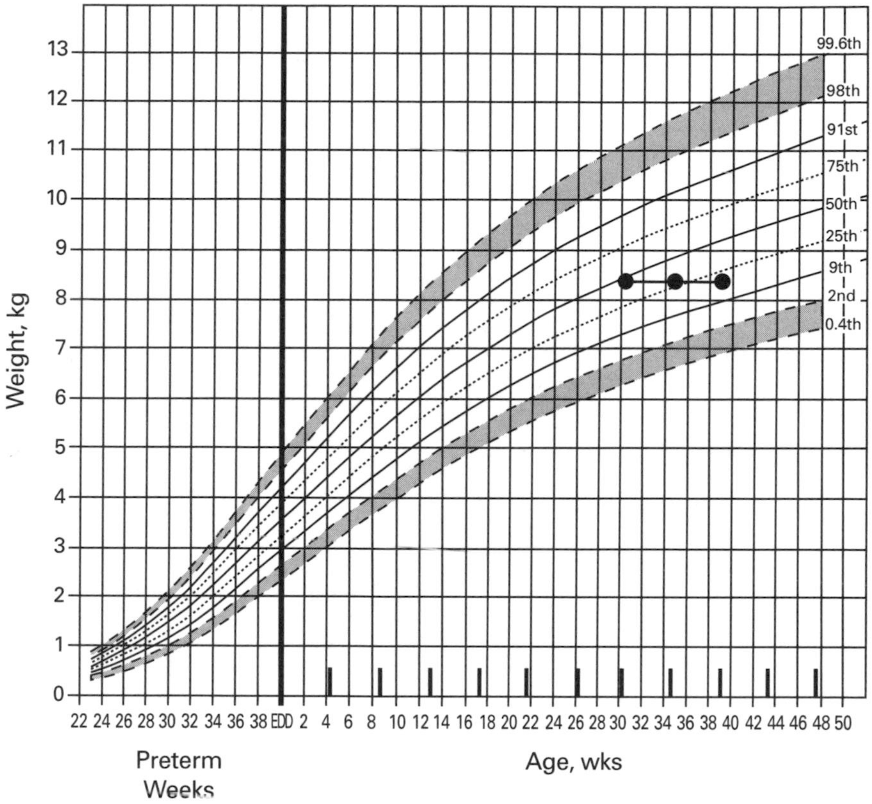

Reprinted with permission from the Child Growth Foundation.

Growth Standards

National reference charts such as the British 1990 or US CDC 2000 indicate how an average child is expected to grow. However, there is no implication that the pattern of growth they represent is any sense *optimal*, it is just *average*. A growth "standard," in contrast, is a growth reference based on a population that has been selected to grow "optimally," so it represents a pattern of growth that children can be encouraged to follow. Children who are likely to grow optimally, and thus who can be used to construct a growth standard, include those who are breastfed or are infants of nonsmoking mothers or of parents in a high socioeconomic class.

Figure 2. The British Breast-from-Birth boys weight chart from birth to 12 months, based on the growth of breastfed infants.[10]

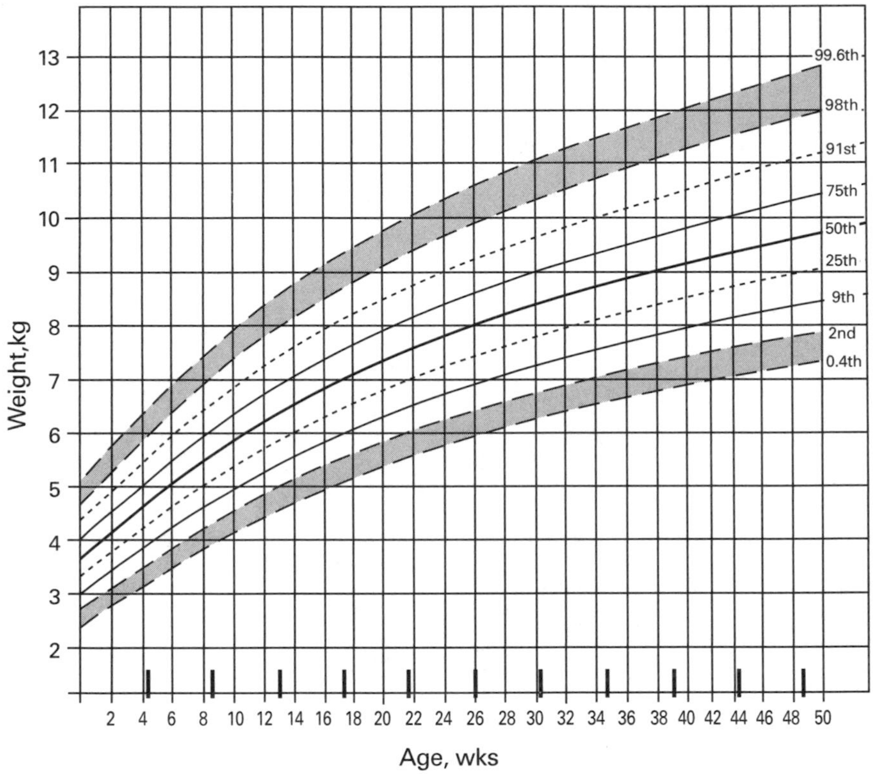

Reprinted with permission from the Child Growth Foundation.

The United Kingdom has had a weight chart for breastfed infants (versus bottlefed infants) for some 3 years (see Figure 2).[10] This chart is based on the typical growth pattern of breastfed infants: which is, rapid growth in the first 2 months of life, followed by slower growth in the latter half of the first year. The chart establishes slower growth later as the norm. Therefore, when healthcare professionals use it, they are less likely to encourage mothers who are breastfeeding their infants to switch to formula feeding so their infants grow faster.[11]

In April 2006 the World Health Organization (WHO) published its long-awaited child growth standard,[12] and this will radically alter the climate of infant weight assessment. Covering the age range 0 to 5 years, the WHO standard is based on infants of mothers who were nonsmokers, from a high socioeconomic class, and followed the WHO and United Nations Children's Emergency Fund (UNICEF) infant feeding guidelines. The mothers and their infants were recruited from sites in 6 countries (Brazil, Ghana, India, Norway, Oman and the United States). The expectation was that growth in these infants is close to optimal, and hence will be very similar from country to country. The WHO standard is likely to be adopted for routine use in many countries, including some countries that already have their own national growth references, and so its impact on growth assessment will be considerable.

Growth Velocity and Thrive Lines

Growth charts are used throughout the world to assess the nutritional status of infants and children, but, they cannot assess growth velocity. They indicate whether a child is large or small, or tall or short, at any given age, as quantified by their corresponding centile. A child who tracks along the centiles over time shows average growth (ie, median growth velocity). However, growth velocity, which involves centile change over time, or centile crossing, is visible qualitatively on the chart but is not quantified in any way. The chart fails to indicate whether or not the rate of centile crossing is excessive — either up or down. This is a significant, but not widely understood failure of the growth chart. It requires considerable expertise to know whether a child's weight that falls by 1 channel width on the growth chart — which is the gap between 2 centiles — is of concern or not, and to understand how the assessment and conclusion varies according to a child's age.

For example, consider the infant's growth pattern illustrated in Figure 1. The chart shows in 2 distinct ways that this infant has grown poorly from 7 to 9 months of age: He did not gain any weight during this 2-month time period, and his weight centile fell by slightly more than 1 channel width. His weight velocity is clearly below the median. But the key question, which is not answered by the chart, is: Should this pattern of growth be a cause for concern? Healthcare providers cannot glean from the chart just how often a pattern as this occurs. Is it within the 1st or the 30th weight velocity centile? These centiles have very different implications in terms of management of an infant's feeding.

The correct and accurate way to assess an infant's weight velocity is to use a velocity chart. Velocity charts are available for weight in infancy[13] or height in childhood,[14] but they are specialist tools used rarely outside the growth clinic. There are several reasons for this:

- A suitable velocity chart may not exist. For example, many European countries have charts for height distance but not height velocity
- The child's growth needs to be measured at regular intervals (eg, annually for height); measurements collected outside this regime cannot be assessed
- The velocities need to be calculated by taking the difference between adjacent measurements and dividing by the time interval between them
- The chart does not adjust for regression to the mean (ie, the fact that smaller babies tend to grow faster)
- Velocities must be plotted on the velocity chart. Therefore, healthcare providers must do twice the amount of plotting and maintain 2 charts rather than just 1

A different approach to monitoring weight velocity is to quantify the degree of centile crossing on the standard growth chart. Remember that tracking along the centiles corresponds to average growth (ie, median growth velocity). It is possible to work out the degree of centile crossing as it corresponds to centiles of growth velocity (eg, the 5th or 95th velocity centile)[15] by using thrive lines. Thrive lines are a set of lines, available on a transparent plastic overlay, that are placed on top of the weight chart and indicate the amount of centile crossing corresponding to the 5th weight velocity centile over a 4-week period.[16] An infant whose weight gain shows greater centile crossing downward over this period than indicated by the thrive lines has a weight velocity below the 5th weight velocity centile. Furthermore, if the growth curve continues to follow this pattern for more than 4 weeks, then the corresponding weight velocity centile is even smaller. For example, tracking in this downward pattern along the thrive lines for 8 weeks corresponds roughly to the 1st velocity centile, which is a more extreme drop in weight velocity than following the same downward pattern over a 4-week period.

Figure 3. The British 1990 boys weight chart from birth to 12 months, for a hypothetical child weighed at 7, 8 and 9 months of age, as shown in Figure 1, with the addition of the 5th centile thrive lines.

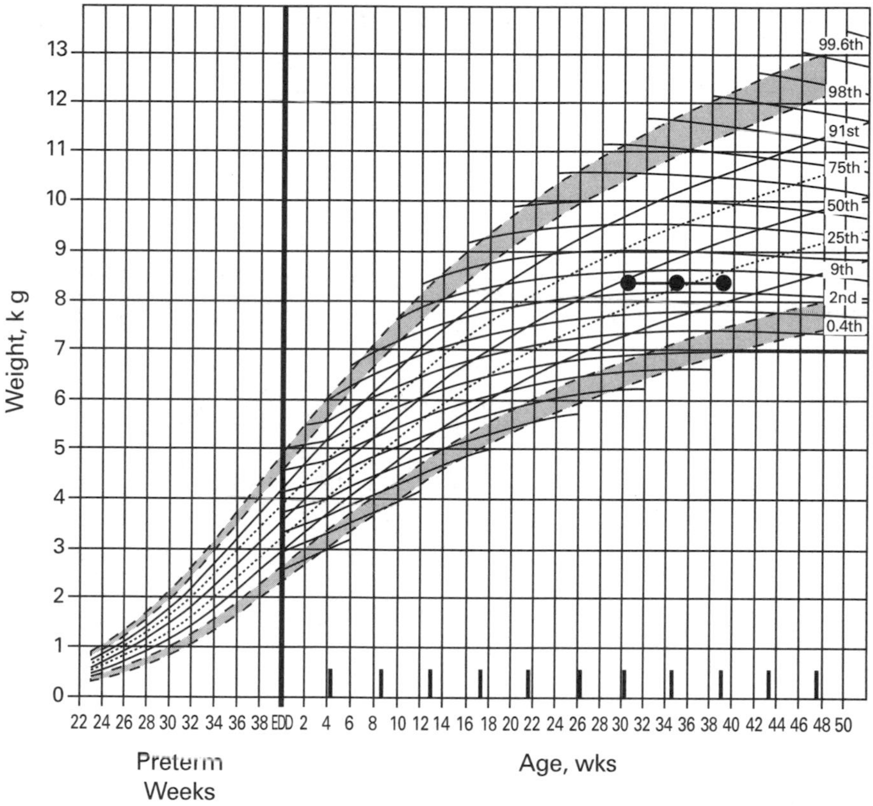

Reprinted with permission from the Child Growth Foundation.

Figure 3 shows the addition of thrive lines to the growth chart in Figure 1. When looking at the augmented growth chart, a healthcare provider can discern whether a child's growth curve: (a) tracks along the thrive lines; (b) crosses thrive lines upward; or (c) crosses thrive lines downward.

Option (a) corresponds to the 5th weight velocity centile, option (b) to a weight velocity above the 5th centile and option (c) to a weight velocity below the 5th centile. In fact, in Figure 3 the child is growing parallel to the thrive lines, at both 7 and 8 months of age. At 7 months of age, the child's growth curve shows a weight velocity on the 5th centile, indicating that 5% of babies grow more slowly than this. At 8 months of age, this continued growth pattern is more extreme and corresponds to the 1st velocity centile, indicating that only 1% of babies grow more slowly than this.

In this example, what appears to be an extreme pattern of growth (the hypothetical child gains no weight over a 2-month period) is seen to be fairly common at this age for the first month (some 5% of infants who are 7 months of age grow more slowly than this), while the continuation of no weight gain into a second month is a rarer event and a matter of concern. Without the thrive lines, a healthcare provider could not make this assessment. Thus, thrive lines are a practical addition to the growth chart as they compensate for the chart's main inadequacy, an inability to highlight patterns of growth velocity that are a concern.

Adjusting Height Based on Family History

During infancy, weight is the growth measurement of choice because it is relatively easy to obtain, and reflects the overall health of the child. An infant's length, in contrast, is difficult to measure accurately. After infancy, however, the measurement of choice shifts from weight to height, which can be accurately measured at 2 years of age or earlier, if the child is able to stand comfortably.

Height charts are a useful tool for identifying children who are unusually short or tall. As described earlier, the British 1990 growth chart has an extra centile, the 0.4th centile, which identifies the shortest 4 children per 1000 children; there is a clear recommendation that healthcare providers refer any child below the 0.4th centile (or, equivalently, above the 99.6th centile) for further consultation.[17]

A 2001 Dutch study showed that this screening process is improved if the height of the child's parents is taken into account.[18] Adjusting for parental height increases the likelihood that healthcare professionals will uncover a growth issue if a child is short but has relatively tall parents. This height adjustment is even more effective if it is extended beyond parents to include one or more of the child's siblings.[19]

The underlying principle is this: If a child has a growth disorder, the family's height is a better proxy than the child's own height for his or her future height potential. Thus, if a child is treated with growth hormone, the family height gives an indication how tall he/she may grow. Conversely, if the child does not have a growth disorder, his or her own height — and the trend over time — are better predictors of future height potential.[18]

Assessment of Adiposity

Weight and height charts indicate the child's size, but the current public health concern is obesity, which relates more directly to a child's shape. After infancy, weight charts are of little value, and measures of shape reflecting adiposity are increasingly important. Adiposity is difficult to measure directly, but healthcare professionals have traditionally used indices of weight adjusted for height as a proxy for fatness.[20] The most commonly used is the body mass index or BMI (weight/height^2),[21] and national BMI charts now exist for several countries.[6,22,23] The median BMI curve, unlike median weight or height, increases steeply during infancy and peaks at 8 to 9 months of age; it subsequently falls slightly, then rises a second time — which is the adiposity rebound[24] — at about 6 years of age and continues to rise until adulthood.

BMI is a simple and broadly effective measure of adiposity, but it has one major weakness — it fails to differentiate between fat mass and fat-free mass.[25] Interventions to prevent or manage obesity often involve a 2-pronged attack to encourage healthy eating and increase physical activity, and they can have opposite effects on BMI. Healthy eating aims to reduce fat mass, while exercise increases muscle mass. Therefore, an effective dual intervention may actually have little impact on BMI because the effects of these 2 different strategies cancel each other out. For this reason, indirect measures of body composition, such as waist circumference (a proxy for abdominal fat)[26] or bioelectric impedance analysis[27] (which approximates fat-free mass), are useful additions to BMI in assessing adiposity. Simple measures of fat mass are notoriously imprecise and inaccurate,[28,29] and the ultimate, easily used population-based measure of body composition has yet to be discovered.

Prediction of Later Size

As discussed previously, a child's size in late childhood or adulthood can be predicted from his or her size at an earlier age, and the child's own size is a better predictor than the size of their parents or other family members (for a child without a growth problem). In general, the shorter the time interval between the predicted growth and the expected height or weight outcome, the more accurate the prediction is — and children on a high and/or rising centile are more likely to be large (ie, on a high centile) than their smaller or slower-growing peers. The reverse holds true for children on a low and/or falling centile: They are likely to be smaller (ie, on a low centile) than their taller or faster-growing peers.[30] This follows a horse racing principle that states that at any point in a horse race, horses that are nearer to the front and/or overtaking other horses are the most likely to win.

Predicting Height in Children and Adolescents

Growth tends to track steadily after infancy; that is, once children have settled into a growth centile, they tend to stay there. This is particularly true for height; year-on-year correlations of height centile during childhood before puberty are well above 0.98.[31] Weight tracks slightly less strongly, and BMI slightly less than weight. Even so, birth weight is a significant predictor of adult weight, and it is possible to predict a child's adult height from their length beginning as early as 9 months of age. Before 9 months of age, length shows considerable centile crossing, which weakens its predictive value. The confidence interval around the height prediction narrows as the child gets older, but widens again during puberty when the variable timing of the pubertal growth spurt weakens the correlation.[3]

Predicting Body Mass Index

Predicting obesity in individual children is an important public health objective; however, there is some debate about the value of implementing a formal obesity screening program. A child's age at adiposity rebound has been found to be weakly predictive of being overweight later in life. Specifically, adiposity rebound at an earlier age is predictive of a higher BMI in late childhood, adolescence and/or adulthood.[24] A higher BMI at the age at adiposity rebound is also a marker for later overweight.[30]

The age at adiposity rebound reflects the child's pattern of BMI centile change at that age; an earlier age at rebound corresponds to a rising BMI centile. Thus a child with a high BMI and an early rebound has a high and rising BMI centile.[30] According to the horse racing principle, this hypothetical child is more likely to track on a high BMI centile later in childhood. Thrive lines can also be used to detect excessive growth in infancy, defined as a growth rate exceeding the 95th weight velocity centile over a 4-week period.[15]

Early Growth and Later Outcomes

For a long time, the pattern of prenatal and infant growth was primarily a clinical concern. Then in the 1980s, the Fetal Origins of Adult Disease (FOAD) hypothesis, proposed by Barker, shifted the onus firmly to public health.[32] Barker's hypothesis was that poor prenatal growth — caused by maternal malnutrition and flagged by low birth weight — programmed the child to be at risk of developing chronic disease in later life. The basis for their hypothesis was the observation of inverse correlations between birth weight and adult diseases such as heart disease, stroke and type 2 diabetes mellitus.

The Barker hypothesis has evolved, and is now called the Developmental Origins of Health and Disease (DOHaD) hypothesis. In its new form, the DOHaD hypothesis reflects the realization that low birth weight is correlated with rapid weight gain after birth, and that it may be this rapid weight gain, rather than the low birth weight, that relates to later poor health outcomes.[33] Indeed, there is growing evidence that rapid infant weight gain is a potent risk factor for poor health outcomes in childhood and adulthood, including obesity,[34-37] insulin resistance[38-40] and elevated blood pressure.[41-43]

A recent paper synthesizes these observations and proposes a "growth acceleration" hypothesis, suggesting that rapid weight gain early in life is a risk factor for adverse health outcomes later in life.[44] One of the most interesting aspects of this hypothesis is the question of the likely direction of causation in the link between weight gain and diet: Does rapid weight gain lead to an increase in dietary intake or, conversely, does increased intake drive rapid weight gain? Or perhaps something else entirely is driving both?

Early Growth, Appetite and Ghrelin

It is possible that increased appetite in a child soon after birth drives both food intake and growth. If this were true, that appetite underlies the growth acceleration hypothesis, it immediately raises the question: Why? One possible explanation is that in the current obesogenic environment, a child with a large appetite is more likely to be fed the sorts of energy-dense foods that are now widespread, whereas a less hungry child is not exposed to these foods in the same way. Another possible explanation, which has rather different public health implications, is that infants with a large appetite are programmed that way in utero, most likely because they have an overweight mother (and possibly an overweight father, too).[45]

The recently discovered hormone ghrelin[46] is a marker of appetite. Ghrelin is negatively correlated with birth weight[47] and positively correlated with early weight gain.[48] Thus, low-birth-weight infants, who are programmed to grow relatively fast, have high ghrelin levels, as do other infants who grow rapidly. Ghrelin may be the heretofore missing factor that links dietary intake to growth rate via appetite, and it may also be relevant to the DOHaD debate.

Birth Weight Programs Later Lean Mass

Earlier sections of this chapter may appear contradictory because on the one hand, birth weight is positively correlated with later BMI (high birth weight predicts high BMI later in life), while on the other hand, low birth weight is associated with later obesity and other adverse health outcomes.[32] However, these apparent contradictions can be explained by differences in body composition. Birth weight is a predictor of later lean mass: High birth weight predicts high lean mass.[49] Lean mass (sometimes called fat-free mass) is 1 component of body weight; the other is fat mass. When lean mass is increased, it affects BMI but not adiposity. Increases in weight after birth, particularly later in childhood, result in greater increases in fat mass than in lean mass, in turn affecting both BMI and adiposity.[49]

Conclusions

Growth assessment — including the nutrition and diet of infants and children — is an essential part of pediatrics. Growth is an indicator of the current health status of the child, predicts future size, and is a risk factor for adult health outcomes and longevity.

References

1. Whitehead RG, Paul AA, Cole TJ. Diet and the growth of healthy infants. *Journal of Human Nutrition and Dietetics.* 1989;2:73-84.
2. Davis JA, Dobbing J, eds. *Scientific Foundations of Pediatrics.* London, England; Heinemann Medical; 1974.
3. Tanner JM. *Growth at Adolescence.* 2nd ed. Oxford: Blackwell, England; 1962.
4. Cole TJ. The use and construction of anthropometric growth reference standards. *Nutrition Research Reviews.* 1993;6:19-50.
5. Freeman JV, Cole TJ, Chinn S, Jones PRM, White EM, Preece MA. Cross sectional stature and weight reference curves for the UK, 1990. *Archives of Disease in Childhood.* 1995;73:17-24.
6. Ogden CL, Kuczmarski RJ, Flegal KM, et al. Centers for Disease Control and Prevention 2000 growth charts for the United States: improvements to the 1977 National Center for Health Statistics version. *Pediatrics.* 2002;109:45-60.
7. Fredriks AM, van Buuren S, Burgmeijer RJ, et al. Continuing positive secular growth change in The Netherlands 1955-1997. *Pediatric Research.* 2000;47:316-323.
8. Cole TJ, Green PJ. Smoothing reference centile curves: the LMS method and penalized likelihood. *Statistics in Medicine.* 1992;11:1305-1319.
9. Cole TJ. Do growth chart centiles need a face lift? *British Medical Journal.* 1994;308:641-642.
10. Cole TJ, Paul AA, Whitehead RG. Weight reference charts for British long-term breastfed infants. *Acta Paediatrica.* 2002;91:1296-1300.
11. Williams AF. Growth charts for breastfed babies. *Acta Paediatrica.* 2002;91:1282-1283.
12. de Onis M, Garza C, Onyango AW, Martorell R. WHO child growth standards. *Acta Paediatrica.* 2006;95 (suppl 450):3-101
13. Roche AF, Guo S, Moore WM. Weight and recumbent length from 1 to 12 mo of age: reference data for 1-mo increments. *American Journal of Clinical Nutrition.* 1989;49:599-607.
14. Tanner JM. Some notes on the recording of growth data. *Human Biology.* 1951;23:93-159.
15. Cole TJ. Presenting information on growth distance and conditional velocity in one chart: practical issues of chart design. *Statistics in Medicine.* 1998;17:2697-2707.
16. Cole TJ. 3-in-1 weight monitoring chart [research letter]. *Lancet.* 1997;349:102-103.
17. Hall DMB. *Health for All Children.* 4th ed. Oxford, England: Oxford University Press; 2003.
18. van Buuren S, Fredriks M. Worm plot: a simple diagnostic device for modelling growth reference curves. *Statistics in Medicine.* 2001;20:1259-1277.
19. Cole TJ. A simple chart to assess non-familial short stature. *Archives of Disease in Childhood.* 2000;82:173-176.
20. Cole TJ. Weight-stature indices to measure underweight, overweight and obesity. In: Himes JH, ed. *Anthropometric Assessment of Nutritional Status.* New York, NY: Wiley-Liss; 1991:83-111.

21. Dietz WH, Robinson TN. Use of the body mass index (BMI) as a measure of overweight in children and adolescents. *Journal of Pediatrics.* 1998;132:191-193.
22. Cole TJ, Freeman JV, Preece MA. Body mass index reference curves for the UK, 1990. *Archives of Disease in Childhood.* 1995;73:25-29.
23. Fredriks AM, van Buuren S, Wit JM, Verloove Vanhorick SP. Body mass index measurements in 1996-1997 compared with 1980. *Archives of Disease in Childhood.* 2000;82:107-112.
24. Rolland-Cachera MF, Deheeger M, Bellisle F, Sempé M, Guilloud-Bataille M, Patois E. Adiposity rebound in children: a simple indicator for predicting obesity. *American Journal of Clinical Nutrition.* 1984;39:129-135.
25. Treuth MS, Butte NF, Wong WW, Ellis KJ. Body composition in prepubertal girls: comparison of six methods. *International Journal of Obesity and Related Metabolic Disorders.* 2001;25:1352-1359.
26. McCarthy HD, Jarrett KV, Crawley HF. The development of waist circumference percentiles in British children aged 5.0-16.9 years. *European Journal of Clinical Nutrition.* 2001;55:902-907.
27. Pietrobelli A, Andreoli A, Cervelli V, Carbonelli MG, Peroni DG, De Lorenzo A. Predicting fat-free mass in children using bioimpedance analysis. *Acta Diabetologica.* 2003;40:S212-S215.
28. Parker L, Reilly JJ, Slater C, Wells JCK, Pitsiladis Y. Validity of six field and laboratory methods for measurement of body composition in boys. *Obesity Research.* 2003;11:852-858.
29. Elberg J, McDuffie JR, Sebring NG, et al. Comparison of methods to assess change in children's body composition. *American Journal of Clinical Nutrition.* 2004;80:64-69.
30. Cole TJ. Children grow and horses race: is the adiposity rebound a critical period for later obesity? *BMC Pediatrics.* 2004;4:6.
31. Bailey BJR. Monitoring the heights of prepubertal children by the use of standard charts. *Annals of Human Biology.* 1994;21:1-11.
32. Barker DJP. *Mothers, Babies and Health in Later Life.* Edinburgh, Scotland: Churchill Livingstone; 1998.
33. Lucas A, Cole TJ, Gore SM, et al. Multicentre clinical trial of diets for low birthweight infants: interim analysis of short term clinical and biochemical effects of diet [abstract]. *Pediatric Research.* 1984;18:803.
34. Gunnarsdottir I, Thorsdottir I. Relationship between growth and feeding in infancy and body mass index at the age of 6 years. *International Journal of Obesity.* 2003;27:1523-1527.
35. Ong KKL, Ahmed ML, Emmett PM, Preece MA, Dunger DB. Association between postnatal catch-up growth and obesity in childhood: prospective cohort study. *British Medical Journal.* 2000;320:967-971.
36. Stettler N, Kumanyika SK, Katz SH, Zemel BS, Stallings VA. Rapid weight gain during infancy and obesity in young adulthood in a cohort of African Americans. *American Journal of Clinical Nutrition.* 2003;77:1374-1378.
37. Yanovski JA. Rapid weight gain during infancy as a predictor of adult obesity. *American Journal of Clinical Nutrition.* 2003;77:1350-1351.
38. Wilkin TJ, Metcalf BS, Murphy MJ, Kirkby J, Jeffery AN, Voss LD. The relative contributions of birth weight, weight change, and current weight to insulin resistance in contemporary 5-year-olds — the EarlyBird study. *Diabetes.* 2002;51:3468-3472.
39. Soto N, Bazaes RA, Pena V, et al. Insulin sensitivity and secretion are related to catch-up growth in small-for-gestational-age infants at age 1 year: results from a prospective cohort. *Journal of Clinical Endocrinology and Metabolism.* 2003;88:3645-3650.
40. Ong KK, Potau N, Petry CJ, et al. Opposing influences of prenatal and postnatal weight gain on adrenarche in normal boys and girls. *Journal of Clinical Endocrinology and Metabolism.* 2004; 89:2647-2651.
41. Adair LS, Cole TJ. Faster child growth increases risk of high blood pressure in adolescent boys who were thin at birth. *Hypertension.* 2003;41:451-456.

42. Horta B, Barros FC, Victora CG, Cole TJ. Early and late growth and blood pressure in adolescence. *Journal of Epidemiology and Community Health.* 2003;57:226-230.
43. Singhal A, Cole TJ, Lucas A. Early nutrition in preterm infants and later blood pressure: two cohorts after randomised trials. *Lancet.* 2001;357:413-419.
44. Singhal A, Lucas A. Early origins of cardiovascular disease: is there a unifying hypothesis? *Lancet.* 2004;363:1642-1645.
45. Buchan IE, Bundred PE, Kitchiner DJ, Cole TJ. Tall stature is now a risk factor for obesity in three year olds: serial cross-sectional surveys 1988-2003. *International Journal of Obesity.* 2006. In press.
46. Kojima M, Hosoda H, Date Y, Nakazato M, Matsuo H, Kangawa K. Ghrelin is a growth-hormone-releasing acylated peptide from stomach. *Nature.* 1999;402:656-660.
47. Ng PC, Lee CH, Lam CWK, Chan IHS, Wong E, Fok TF. Ghrelin in preterm and term newborns: relation to anthropometry, leptin and insulin. *Clinical Endocrinology.* 2005;63:217-222.
48. James RJA, Drewett RF, Cheetham TD. Low cord ghrelin levels in term infants are associated with slow weight gain over the first 3 months of life. *Journal of Clinical Endocrinology and Metabolism.* 2004;89:3847-3850.
49. Singhal A, Wells J, Cole TJ, Fewtrell M, Lucas A. Programming of lean body mass: a link between birth weight, obesity, and cardiovascular disease? *American Journal of Clinical Nutrition.* 2003;77:726-730.

Obesity in Young Children

Donna M. Matheson, PhD
Thomas N. Robinson, MD, MPH

Introduction

Over the past 3 decades, the United States and the rest of the world have experienced dramatic increases in obesity in both children and adults.[1] In the United States, the prevalence of obesity among children 6 to 19 years of age (as defined by gender- and age-specific body mass index, or BMI, at or above the 95th percentile on the 2000 Centers for Disease Control and Prevention [CDC] growth charts)[2] increased from 4% during 1971-1974[3] to 16% during 1999-2002.[4,5] The percentage of children in the United States 6 to 19 years of age considered overweight (as defined by gender- and age-specific BMI at or above the 85th percentile on the 2000 CDC growth charts) was 31% during 1999-2002.[5] Trends among adults are similar. Between the time periods 1976-1980 and 1999-2002, obesity (defined as BMI $\geq$ 30 kg/m^2) among adults in the United States more than doubled, increasing from more than 14% to 30%.[6]

There are significant ethnic differences in overweight and obesity. For example, among non-Hispanic black and Mexican American children, the rates of overweight and obesity are higher than in the population as a whole. In the 1999-2002 National Health and Nutrition Examination Survey (NHANES), 35% and 21% of non-Hispanic black children and 40% and 22% of Mexican American children had BMI at or above the 85th and 95th percentiles, respectively, on the 2000 CDC growth charts.[5] Furthermore, 10 years earlier, in the 1988-1994 NHANES III, the BMI of non-Hispanic black girls and Mexican American boys and girls 6 to 9 years of age were already beginning to deviate from the BMI of white children of the same age, and this deviation continued to widen throughout later childhood and into young adulthood.[7] Among girls, the racial/ethnic differences in BMI were independent of socioeconomic status.[7] Similar racial/ethnic differences are seen in adults, with non-Hispanic black and Mexican American women having the highest rates of overweight and obesity.[5]

Increases in the prevalence of overweight and obesity have been accompanied by increases in the mean BMI in the population; the degree of increase is not identical across all age groups.[6] Among younger children — 6 to 11 years of age — and to a lesser extent among adolescents, comparisons of BMI distributions in national surveys from the 1960s with BMI distributions from the 1988-1994 NHANES III indicate that the greatest changes in BMI are at the upper end of the BMI distribution, with fewer changes at the lower end. Among adults, comparisons of BMI distributions from the 1976-1980 NHANES II and the 1988-1994 NHANES III show an upward skewing of the mean BMI score, combined with increases in BMI throughout the entire distribution. These findings are expected given that a number of environmental factors act upon the entire population, but the effects may be particularly potent in genetically susceptible groups.[6]

These trends in overweight and obesity have important implications for the health of the population. Obese adults suffer from higher rates of type 2 diabetes mellitus, hypertension, cardiovascular disease, osteoarthritis and cancer.[8] Obesity in children is associated with a host of health problems, including glucose intolerance, type 2 diabetes, hypertension, dyslipidemia, hepatic steatosis, cholelithiasis, sleep apnea, menstrual abnormalities, impaired balance and orthopedic problems.[9] Notably, the recent and rapid rise in the incidence of type 2 diabetes among young children has serious short- and long-term implications for children's health. Since 1990, up to 45% of all newly diagnosed cases of pediatric diabetes have been type 2 diabetes, compared to only 4% of cases diagnosed prior to that time.[10] Accordingly, estimates of the number of young children who will be diagnosed with diabetes at some point in their lives run as high as 30% for boys and 40% for girls.[11] The long-term effects of childhood obesity carry significant costs for society, among them lost productivity, disability, morbidity and premature death.[12]

The childhood obesity rate does not appear to have reached a plateau, thus effective methods to prevent and control childhood overweight are critically needed. Presently, much less is known about the causes, correlates and consequences of overweight among young children than among school-aged children, adolescents and adults. Because nearly one-third of children as young as 6 to 11 years of age in the United States are overweight or obese,[5] prevention and control interventions should begin during early childhood.

Measurement of Overweight in Young Children

Obesity is typically defined as an excess of body fat that is associated with adverse health outcomes. For practical purposes, body weight is measured relative to height to assess obesity in both children and adults. Height and weight can be measured easily, and with a high degree of accuracy and reliability.[13] Body mass index, defined as weight in kilograms divided by the square of height in meters, or kg/m^2, is the most appropriate measure of overweight in children based on its accessibility, individuality (referring to its usefulness for tracking over time), reliability, validity and most importantly, its clinical validity.[14] However, in children, BMI covaries with height. Data from the Bogalusa Heart Study revealed that childhood height at age 5 was independently correlated with adult BMI ($r = 0.41$),[15] and the correlation between the height-for-age percentile of children 2 to 5 years of age and their BMI was 0.29.[16] Moreover, at similar BMI and weight percentiles, children whose height was greater than the 95th percentile were estimated to have a BMI that averaged 1.4 units higher in adulthood than did children at the 50th percentile for height.[16] Nonetheless, it is generally agreed that BMI is the best available measure of adiposity for research, clinical practice and surveillance.[14,17-23]

Different Charts, Different Cut-Off Points Used to Define Obesity

There is less agreement regarding the most appropriate comparison standard and cut-off points to define obesity in children. In 2000, 2 new growth references were released: the CDC 2000 growth charts (http://www.cdc.gov/growthcharts/)[2] and the International Obesity Taskforce (IOTF) growth standards.[18] Prior to the year 2000, National Center for Health Statistics (NCHS) growth charts, based on data from NHANES I and the Fels Research Institute, were used as a reference to define overweight in the United States.[24]

The CDC 2000 growth charts are based on data from NHANES I, II and III. Data collected from children 6 years of age and older in NHANES III were not included in the charts — in order to avoid an upward shift of the weight and BMI curves. However, NHANES III data from preschool-aged children were included.[2] Therefore (compared to school-aged children and adolescents), fewer preschool-aged children may be classified as obese because the BMI range included in the charts may be skewed to the right. On the CDC 2000 growth charts, for children 2 to 5 years of age, as with older children, overweight and obesity are defined as gender- and age-specific BMI at or above the 85th percentile and 95th percentile, respectively.

The IOTF charts — which are based on data from the United States, Great Britain, Brazil, Hong Kong, the Netherlands and Singapore — use adult BMI cut-off points of 25 and 30 to develop corresponding percentiles for children from birth to 18 years of age.[18] For young children 2 to 5 years of age, the cut-off points are higher on the IOTF chart than they are on the CDC 2000 growth charts. Therefore, using the IOTF charts, fewer children are classified as overweight or obese. Based on NHANES III data (1988-1994), a 2001 study confirmed that the prevalence of overweight among youth using the CDC growth charts was higher than the prevalence rates estimated using the IOTF cut-off points.[25] However, longitudinal data from children 4 to 15 years of age who participated in the Bogalusa Heart Study and were followed for another 13 to 24 years revealed that the cut-off points for overweight based on the CDC 2000 growth charts and the IOTF BMI references nearly equally predicted adult obesity, abdominal obesity, hypertension, high LDL cholesterol, low HDL cholesterol, high triglycerides and metabolic syndrome.[26] The cut-offs from the CDC reference were slightly more sensitive but less specific than the IOTF cut-off points (as would be expected based on the differences noted earlier). As a result, some individual children may be classified differently by the 2 references. Nonetheless, both the CDC 2000 growth charts and the IOTF BMI reference appear to be appropriate references for public health surveillance.[26]

Trends in BMI and Prevalence of Overweight in Young Children

The anthropometric measures and growth patterns of preschool-aged children have been described in a number of cross-sectional and longitudinal studies. In the United States, the NHANES and the CDC Pediatric Nutrition Surveillance System (PedNSS) — which includes children enrolled in the Women, Infants, and Children program (WIC), and other publicly funded health programs for children — are the primary sources of data used to document the prevalence of overweight and obesity in preschool-aged children (2 to 5 years of age).

- The most recent cycle of NHANES data collection in 1999-2002 included 1522 children 2 to 5 years of age of the following ethnic composition: 30% non-Hispanic white, 29% non-Hispanic black, 31% Mexican American, and 10% Asian, Pacific Islanders and others.
  - In this sample, 23% of children had BMI above the 85th percentile, and 10% of children had BMI above the 95th percentile on the CDC 2000 growth charts.[5]
  - In this age group, there were no statistically significant gender or racial/ethnic differences in the prevalence rates for overweight or obesity.[3,5]
- Examination of previous NHANES data collection cycles (NHANES II: 1976-1980 and III: 1988-1994; n = 7480) revealed that over the past 25 years, the number of preschool-aged children classified as overweight has doubled.[3]
  - In comparison to the 1999-2002 NHANES data reported above, NHANES III data (1988-1994) indicated that only 11% of children 2 to 5 years of age had BMI above the 85th percentile and just 8% of children had BMI above the 95th percentile on the CDC 2000 growth charts.[27]
  - Among boys, racial/ethnic differences in obesity rates were consistent across the NHANES 1999-2000[3] and NHANES III[28] samples. At all ages, the number of Hispanic boys above the 95th percentile on the 2000 CDC growth charts (NHANES 1999-2000 sample) and the 95th percentile on the NCHS weight-for-stature charts (based on the NHANES III sample) was higher than it was for either their non-Hispanic white or black counterparts.[3,28]
  - In contrast, among girls, racial/ethnic differences in obesity prevalence rates varied by sample: The number of girls above the 95th percentile on the CDC 2000 growth charts was higher for Hispanics than it was for non-Hispanic blacks or whites in the NHANES III 1988-1994 sample, but in the NHANES 1999-2000 sample, non-Hispanic black girls were more likely to be above the 95th percentile on the NCHS weight-for-stature charts than were the other 2 ethnic groups. These trends remained even when the NHANES 1988-1994 data were adjusted for gestational weight and body proportion (assessed by the

ratio of sitting height to standing height). The BMI of non-Hispanic black children increased when adjusted for body proportionality, resulting in BMI that were closer to the BMI of Hispanic children.[29]

- The prevalence rates of obesity for preschool-aged girls differed from those of preschool-aged boys. In general, girls of all ages were significantly more likely than boys to be obese, as defined by measurements at or above the 95th percentile on the NCHS weight-for-stature charts.[28] Among girls, both overweight (defined as being between the 85th and 94th percentile on the CDC 2000 growth charts) and obesity (defined as being above the 95th percentile) increased between 3 and 5 years of age. Among the boys, the prevalence of overweight increased between 3 and 4 years of age, but decreased between 4 and 5 years of age. The opposite pattern was observed for obesity among boys: The prevalence of obesity decreased between 3 and 4 years of age, but increased between 4 and 5 years of age.[27]
- The obesity epidemic in preschool-aged children is characterized by both an increase in the *prevalence* of obesity and an increase in the *severity* of obesity over time.[30] Severity of obesity is measured by the amount that an obese child exceeds his or her age- and gender-specific 95th percentile cut-off based on the CDC 2000 growth charts. On average, obese preschool-aged children (2 to 5 years of age) exceeded their age- and gender-specific 95th percentiles by 8% in the first NHANES (1971-1974) and by 12% in NHANES III (1988-1994). In the 1999-2000 NHANES, the severity of obesity decreased to 9%. However, this decrease is likely the result of the increase in the overall number of children classified as obese because severity of obesity is adjusted by the prevalence rate.

The Pediatric Nutrition Surveillance System

The PedNSS has been used to examine the prevalence of overweight in low-income children enrolled in public health programs, primarily WIC,[31] and to examine trends in overweight across the 50 states.[32] Collection methods for surveillance data are often not well standardized across sites, and there may be high rates of incomplete data.[33] However, for the PedNSS data collected in 1989, 1994 and 2000, the percent of records with biologically implausible values for weight-for-height (z score < 4 or > 5) was less than 1%,[32] although the validity of the actual height and weight measures were not reported.

- Mei and colleagues examined 15,029,147 PedsNSS records from 1983 to 1995 for children 0 to 5 years of age to assess the prevalence of obesity in this population.[31] Compared to the NHANES II and III samples, the PedNSS samples included more Hispanic and black children; more children living in urban areas and more children with lower birth weights, lower height-for-age and lower weight-for-age *z* scores, but higher weight-for-height *z* scores. In the PedNSS, children were considered obese if they scored higher than the 95th percentile on the NCHS weight-for-height reference charts. Mei and colleagues found that the prevalence of obesity increased from 1983 to 1995 in both boys and girls across all ethnicities and all ages. Obesity was highest in Hispanics, followed by non-Hispanic blacks, and was lowest among non-Hispanic whites ($P<.05$). Prevalence rates tended to be higher in children 4 to 5 years of age than in younger children. In addition, the prevalence of obesity was higher among girls than among boys ($P<.05$).[31]

- Sherry and colleagues[32] used PedNSS records (n = 2,092,444) from 1989, 1994 and 2000 to examine the prevalence of obesity across the states among children 2 to 4 years of age. Obesity was defined as scoring higher than the 95th percentile on the CDC 2000 growth charts. In this study, the researchers found that obesity increased from 11% in 1989 to almost 14% in 2000. Similar to previous reports, obesity increased with age, and Hispanic children had the highest rates of obesity. Contrary to other analyses of NHANES or PedNSS data, Sherry and colleagues reported that boys had a higher prevalence of obesity than girls. Data from the year 2000 revealed that 14% of boys were obese compared to 13% of girls.[32] This discrepancy in results is probably due to differences in the BMI cut-off points used to define overweight. Mei and colleagues used the NCHS growth curves to estimate prevalence rates,[31] while the analysis by Sherry and colleagues used the CDC 2000 growth standards that has BMI cut-off points that are slightly higher than the NCHS cut-off points.[32]

- Most nationally representative samples do not separately examine the prevalence of obesity and overweight for American Indians. However, Sherry and colleagues reported that the prevalence of obesity in American Indian children was second only to Hispanics. PedNSS data from the year 2000 revealed that 17% of American Indian children ranked above the 95th percentile on the CDC 2000 growth charts.[32] In addition, a smaller study (n = 252) of PedNSS records of American Indian children from 1997 to 2001 revealed that the prevalence of obesity among American

Indians was almost double the rate observed among the entire population of children in NHANES III. Nearly 19% of American Indian children 3 years of age were above the 85th percentile on the CDC 2000 growth charts and more than 22% were above the 95th percentile.[34] Other racial/ethnic groups have not been included in sufficient numbers in national surveys to document these trends, although other Hispanic groups, Native Americans, Alaskan Natives and Pacific Islanders have been identified as groups at particularly high risk for obesity.[35,36] More research on obesity among these particularly high-risk populations is needed.

In summary, obesity among preschool-aged children is a well-documented public health crisis. Both NHANES and PedNSS data reveal that at least 10% of the preschool-aged population is obese and approximately 20% is overweight. Similar to what has been seen among older children, adolescents and adults, the prevalence of overweight among children is escalating, with no indication of it leveling off.[5,6]

Tracking Obesity From Young Childhood Through Adolescence and Adulthood: An Overview of Longitudinal Research

A significant body of longitudinal research has tracked children's BMI as they grow to determine whether childhood obesity is associated with obesity in adulthood (see Table 1). Since the 1960s, multiple studies have looked at the association between measures of adiposity in young children, such as BMI or skinfolds, and follow-up measures of adiposity collected in adolescence or adulthood. In these studies, the relative risk of obesity in adulthood when an individual is obese in childhood ranged from 1.1 to 19.3 (see Table 1). The variations in the strength of these associations are related to differences in BMI cut-off points, definitions of obesity, the age of baseline assessment and the length of follow-up.[22] Serdula and colleagues conducted a literature review and identified 9 studies that reported correlations between adiposity in children (6 months of age to 4 years of age) and adiposity in adults that ranged from 0.04 to 0.32. In these studies, 21% to 41% of overweight preschool-aged children were also overweight as adults.[37]

Table 1. Summary of Studies Tracking Childhood Obesity

Reference	Subjects	Obesity Criteria	Baseline Age	Follow-up Age	% Obese at Follow-up	Relative Risk of Adult Obesity
Asher[38] (1966)	n = 137 clinic patients England	wt >90th percentile of the sample distribution	6 m	3-4 y	44%	6.6
Fisch, et al[39] (1975)	n = 1779 infants United States	wt/ht >95th percentile relative to age and sex in the sample distribution	birth	7 y	19%	4.4
Charney, et al[40] (1976)	n = 366 United States	Baseline wt >90th percentile once or more in 1st 6 m vs comparison group with wt between 25th & 75th percentile in 1st 6 m. Follow-up >120% standard wt/ht of the sample	≤6 m	20-30 y		2.6
Johnston & Mack[41] (1978)	n = 798 black children United States	Baseline wt/ht >1 std dev above the sample mean at 1 y. Follow-up triceps skinfold >90th percentile of the sample distribution	1 y	9-15 y	M 42% F 32%	
Zack, et al[42] (1979)	n = 1993 United States	>75th percentile of the sample distribution, sum of triceps & subscapular skinfold thickness for age, sex & race	6-11 y	12-17 y (2-5 y follow-up)	69%	7.3
Stark, et al[43] (1981)	n = 5362 England	>120% average wt/ht for age & sex for children born in 1946 in the National Survey of Health and Human Development	7 y 11 y 14 y 20 y	26 y 26 y 26 y 26 y	42% 40% 50% 75%	4.0
Garn & La Velle[44] (1985)	n = 383 United States	Subscapular or triceps skinfold >85th percentile of the sample distribution	0.5-5 y	19-25 y	26.6%	1.8
Rolland-Cachera, et al[45] (1987)	n = 164 France	BMI >75th percentile of the French reference population	1 y	20-30 y	41%	2.0
Freedman, et al[46] (1987)	n = 1490 United States	Triceps skinfold >85th percentile of the sample distribution	2-14 y (mean 7.3)	10-24 y (mean 15.7)	43%	4.3
Mossberg[47] (1989)	n = 352 Sweden	Baseline wt/ht ≥2 standard deviation above mean. Follow-up wt/ht ≥1 standard deviation above mean (15% >ideal body weight)	0.4-16 yr	20-60 yr	51%	
Muramatsu, et al[48] (1990)	n = 309 males n = 335 females Japan	Wt/ht^2 >90th percentile at birth, 3 y & 17 y of the sample distribution	birth 3 y	17 y 17 y	M 12% F 24% M 30% F 22%	1.1 2.7 3.7 2.3
Prokopec & Bellisle[49] (1993)	n = 80 males n = 78 females Czech	Baseline >75th percentile of the sample distribution at 12 months follow-up	3 m	18 y		1.8
Clarke & Lauer[50] (1993)	n = 2631 United States	Upper quintile of the sample distribution for BMI by age and sex	9-12 y	21-25 y 26-30 y	M 63% F 67% M 64% F 60%	
Gasser, et al[51] (1995)	n = 120 males n = 112 females Switzerland	Upper quintile of the distribution	birth	20 y		M-3 F-2
Guo, et al[52] (2002)	n = 166 males n = 181 females United States	BMI ≥30 BMI ≥72nd percentile at 18 y on CDC 2000 growth charts	3 y	35 y	M 12% F 11%	M 19.3 F 15.7
Freedman, et al[53] (2005)	n = 151 2-5 y boys n = 234 2-5 y girls United States	≥ 85th percentile on CDC 2000 growth chart	2-5 y	19±3 y follow-up	M 20.7% F 27.4%	M 6.4 F 2.9

In the United States, the Bogalusa Heart Study, which collected data between 1976 and 1996, is one of the most comprehensive longitudinal studies of children's adiposity and cardiovascular health.[54] In a sample of 2610 black and white participants, correlations between BMI and tricep skinfolds at 2 to 5 years of age and subsequently as adults were 0.50 for both measures in males and 0.45 for BMI and 0.38 for skinfolds in females. Approximately 73% of girls 2 to 5 years of age with BMI above the 95th percentile on the CDC 2000 growth charts became obese women (BMI ≥ 30). Among boys 2 to 5 years of age, 93% of those with BMI above the 85th percentile on the CDC 2000 growth charts became obese men.[54] (Only 8 preschool-aged boys in the sample had BMI above the 95th percentile on the CDC 2000 growth charts and they were therefore grouped with boys whose BMI were above the 85th percentile on the CDC 2000 growth charts.) In an earlier report of the Bogalusa data, 77% of 186 children with a mean age of 10 years who had BMI above the 95th percentile later became obese adults (BMI ≥ 30), while only 7% of 1317 children with BMI less than the 85th percentile became obese adults.[55] Furthermore, while less than half of the 581 adults in the Bogalusa Heart Study who were obese had BMI above the 85th percentile as children (25% had BMI above the 95th percentile and 22% had BMI between the 85th and 95th percentiles at 10 years of age), obese adults who had also been obese as children had a higher average adult BMI than did obese adults who were not obese as children. The average BMI of adults whose BMI was above the 95th percentile on the CDC 2000 growth charts prior to 8 years of age was 42, compared to an average BMI of 34 in adults whose BMI increased later in childhood or during adolescence.[15]

Tracking BMI and Weight Into Adulthood: Racial, Age and Gender Differences

Differences in how childhood BMI and weight tracks into adulthood by race, age and gender have been observed. Prospective research from the National Longitudinal Survey of Youth (NLSY) conducted between 1986 and 1998 on children 4 to 12 years of age revealed that over time the number of ethnic minority children with BMI above the 95th percentile on the CDC 2000 growth charts increased more rapidly than did the number of non-Hispanic white children, thereby potentially increasing the health inequities between these 2 groups of youth. Specifically, between 1986 and 1998, obesity increased 120% in Hispanic and non-Hispanic black children, but only 50%

in non-Hispanic white children.[56] In the Bogalusa Heart Study, non-Hispanic black girls, regardless of their BMI score, were more likely to become obese women than were their non-Hispanic white counterparts. Approximately 84% of non-Hispanic black girls with BMI above the 95th percentile on the CDC 2000 growth charts became obese (BMI ≥ 30), while 65% of non-Hispanic white girls with BMI above the 95th percentile did so. In a similar vein, 82% of non-Hispanic black boys with BMI above the 95th percentile became obese men compared to 71% of non-Hispanic white boys with BMI above the 95th percentile.[53] Interestingly, non-Hispanic white boys with BMI at or below the 50th percentile on the CDC 2000 growth charts were more likely to become obese or overweight men than were non-Hispanic black boys who ranked at the same place on the growth charts.[53]

The longitudinal relationship between childhood and adult obesity is age related. Obesity in older children is more likely to persist into adulthood than obesity in younger children. A retrospective study in a health maintenance organization found that children 1 to 2 years of age with BMI above the 95th percentile on the CDC 2000 growth charts were not more likely to be obese as adults (BMI ≥ 30).[57] However, by the time children were 3 to 5 years of age, obesity tracked into adulthood: 24% of children with BMI between the 85th and 94th percentiles and 33% of children with BMI above the 95th percentile on the CDC 2000 growth charts became obese adults. In addition, if at least 1 parent was obese, the likelihood of an obese child becoming an obese adult was even greater. Some 62% of children with BMI between the 85th and 94th percentile and 83% of children with BMI above the 95th percentile became obese adults. In this study, there were no gender differences in the probability of childhood overweight persisting into adulthood as overweight or obesity.[57] Conversely, data from the Fels Longitudinal Study[52] revealed that the probability of obesity in preschool-aged children persisting to age 35 differed between boys and girls:

- Some 15% of boys (n = 166) with BMI above the 95th percentile on the CDC 2000 growth charts at 3 years of age, 14% at 4 years of age and 31% at 5 years of age ultimately became obese men (BMI > 30).[52]
- Among girls (n = 181), 24% of those with BMI above the 95th percentile at 3 years of age, 25% at 4 years of age and 37% at 5 years of age later became obese women.[52]

Adiposity/BMI Rebound

Normal growth in preschool-aged children is characterized by a decline in BMI over time. The term adiposity rebound has been used to describe the lowest childhood BMI measurement, which typically occurs between 5 and 7 years of age, and precedes the increase in BMI that continues throughout childhood and adolescence.[58] Early adiposity rebound that occurs prior to 5 to 7 years of age was first found to be associated with higher BMI in adults in a study reported in 1987 of 164 French children followed from 1 month of age to 21 years of age.[45] Subsequently, the relationship between early adiposity rebound and adult obesity was replicated in a number of studies.[52,59-63] Using periodic dual energy X-ray absorptiometry (DXA) scans of 39 girls, a recent study found that the weight gain associated with early adiposity rebound (prior to 5 years of age) may be attributed to increased fat deposition, but not increased lean tissue.[61] By 9 years of age, 3 times as many girls who experienced early adiposity rebound were classified as overweight as compared to their later rebounding peers.[61]

Research has shown that age at adiposity rebound and BMI are highly correlated.[15] Children who have an early adiposity rebound also tend to have higher BMI at 5 years of age.[15,64] However, the relationship between age of adiposity rebound and adult BMI is not significant when adjusted for BMI score at 7 years of age.[15] Therefore, the significance of age at adiposity rebound in determining adult obesity has come under question. The adiposity rebound-adult BMI relationship may also reflect associations between children's BMI prior to rebound and the rate at which their BMI escalates after rebound.[65,66] Furthermore, establishing the exact age of adiposity rebound in a child is difficult and requires multiple measurements around the expected period of adiposity rebound. Therefore, measurement of BMI at 7 years of age may actually be a more practical indicator of the effects of preschool-year growth patterns on obesity later in life.[65,66]

Childhood Obesity and Future Health Risks

Recent research has examined the associations between overweight in children and adult comorbidities, including coronary heart disease, hypertension and diabetes. Most of the findings have not been replicated, and many studies reported relatively weak associations between childhood overweight/obesity and obesity in adulthood.

In a sample of children 5 to 17 years of age from the Bogalusa Heart Study who were followed for an average of 17 years, the researchers reported correlations between adult systolic blood pressure and childhood BMI, as well as fasting serum insulin and childhood BMI of $r = 0.08$ and $r = 0.26$, respectively.[55] However, when adjusted for adult BMI in multivariate analysis, the associations between childhood BMI and adult risk factors were not statistically significant.[55] Another study of the same sample of children from the Bogalusa Heart Study examined carotid intima-media thickness (IMT) in adults relative to childhood and adulthood measurements of BMI.[67] BMI in children under 11 years of age were only moderately associated with adult IMT ($r = 0.12$). However, when adjusted for adult BMI, IMT was significantly associated with childhood BMI only in obese children who subsequently became obese adults. This relationship did not hold for overweight children who were not obese as adults or thinner children who became obese as adults. Therefore, in this sample, childhood obesity that persisted into adulthood appeared to have long-term cumulative effects on cardiovascular health.

Patterns of weight gain in children from birth to 5 years of age have also been found to be associated with cardiovascular disease (CVD) risk factors, including high blood pressure and diabetes. In a retrospective study of 357 men from Helsinki with coronary heart disease, birth records and school examinations showed that those men who had been low-birth-weight infants and experienced rapid catch-up growth during the preschool years were more likely to develop coronary heart disease[68] and high blood pressure.[69] Likewise, in a study of 346 British men and women, low birth weight followed by rapid weight gain between 1 and 5 years of age was associated with higher adult systolic blood pressures.[70] Weight gain prior to 1 year of age was not associated with elevated adult blood pressure. Adult BMI appears to be the mediator in the association between systolic pressure and early childhood weight gain, but does not appear to play such a role in the relationship between birth weight and blood pressure. In the Helsinki sample, rapid weight gain beginning at 2 years of age that was sustained throughout childhood and persisted into the adult years was also associated with the development of type 2 diabetes.[71]

In summary, for many children, overweight during the preschool years tends to persist through adolescence and into adulthood. Moreover, by about 4 years of age, the relationship between weight status and lipoprotein profiles begins to mimic that of adults. In addition, rapid weight gain during the preschool years has been associated with CVD, high blood pressure and type 2 diabetes. These findings indicate that obesity in childhood and adolescence may contribute to the onset of CVD-related risk factors, as well as morbidity and mortality in adulthood.

Obesity in Children and Cardiovascular Risk Factors

CVD risk factors have been studied more than other comorbidities in young children. Analysis of the serum lipids of children enrolled in the Bogalusa Heart Study at birth and followed to 7 years of age revealed that by age 7, children's lipoprotein profiles begin to mimic patterns observed in adults.[72] Children's weight status (measured by Rohrer's Index, weight/height^3) was not associated with serum lipids or lipoproteins for the first 4 years of life, but changes in Rohrer's Index between 6 months of age and 7 years of age were positively associated with changes in triglycerides (TG) and very low-density-lipoprotein cholesterol (VLDL-C).[72] Between 4 and 7 years of age, changes in children's weight status was inversely associated with HDL-C levels.[72] Furthermore, children whose TG, HDL-C and VLDL-C tracked in higher risk categories from 6 months of age to 7 years of age were heavier at age 7 than were children with initial high risk levels that did not continue to track that way over time.

Another analysis from the Bogalusa Heart Study using data on 913 children 5 to 6 years of age found that a BMI above the 95th percentile (calculated using the LMS method and data from Health Examination Survey and NHANES collected between 1963 and 1994) was associated with significantly increased odds (compared to children with a BMI below the 85th percentile) of having TG levels above 130 mg/dL (OR = 7.1), an elevated fasting insulin level (OR = 6.9), and elevated systolic and diastolic blood pressures (OR = 16.0 and 4.8, respectively).[73]

In an autopsy study of children 2 to 15 years of age from Bogalusa, Louisiana, most of the children had fatty streaks in their aortas, approximately 50% had fatty streaks in their coronary arteries, 20% had raised fibrous plaque lesions in their aortas and 8% had these same lesions in their coronary arteries.[74] In addition, among a sample of 93 individuals 2 to 39 years of age (mean age at death was 20.6 years) who had been previously surveyed as part of the Bogalusa Heart Study, BMI prior to their deaths was significantly associated with fatty streaks and fibrous plaques in the aorta (r = 0.33 and r = 0.24, respectively) and the coronary arteries (r = 0.41 and r = 0.29, respectively), and the extent of fatty-streak and fibrous plaque lesions in both the aorta and coronary arteries (r = 0.48).[74]

Associations Between Dietary Intake and Obesity in Preschool Children

Given the potential negative effects that childhood obesity has on both short-term and long-term health, interventions to prevent and control obesity in young children are highly warranted. Children's dietary intake, specifically the macronutrient composition of their diets, has been targeted as one of the factors that may affect children's growth and weight status. Concerns regarding the safety of calorie- and/or fat-reduced diets for young children has led to a considerable amount of research examining the relationships between children's dietary intake, body weight and growth.

Experimental research on the relationship between dietary fat intake and young children's growth was conducted as part of the Special Turku Coronary Risk Factor Intervention Project (STRIP).[75-77] This study involved a sample of 1054 families with children 7 months of age who were randomly assigned to either an experimental group that received nutrition counseling to lower their child's fat intake or to a control group that received no counseling. Nutrition counseling, beginning in infancy, successfully lowered the amount of energy intake that children derived from fat by an average of 2 percentage points at 4 years of age.[75] This decrease in dietary fat intake was maintained until 10 years of age.[76] There were no statistically significant differences between the 2 groups in height, weight or growth velocity from 13 months of age to 5 years of age.[75,77]

This research demonstrated that a childhood diet that derives 25% to 30% of energy intake from fat is compatible with adequate nutrients and normal growth.[75] Furthermore, the lack of a relationship between dietary fat intake and weight is consistent with 2 cross-sectional studies: a sample of predominantly Hispanic children 3 to 4 years of age from the United States[78] and a sample of more than 800 children 3.5 years of age from Great Britain.[79] In both of these studies, the amount of fat in children's diets was not associated with stature, weight status or growth. Although the STRIP intervention was designed to reduce the amount of energy intake children derive from fat through eucaloric diets, children whose parents received the dietary counseling had diets that were slightly lower in energy intake overall (estimated intakes approximately 20-30 kcals/day),[80] and energy intakes were found to be associated with children's weight.[77] Children 3 years of age with weight-for-height scores below the 5th percentile of the Finnish growth references had the lowest energy intakes and children who had weight-for-height scores above the 95th percentile of the Finnish growth reference had the highest daily energy intakes ($P = .024$).[77]

Experimental research to examine the effects of protein intake on weight gain in very young children is lacking. However, some longitudinal studies have examined the associations between protein and fat intake and weight.

The Relationship Between Protein Intake and BMI

- In a sample of 70 white children from mid-socioeconomic status US families, the percent of energy from fat and from protein in children's diets at 2 years of age was weakly associated with BMI at 8 years of age in separate multivariate regression analyses that also included age at adiposity rebound and BMI at 2 years of age.[81]
- Likewise, 2 European studies found weak associations between protein intake at 1 year of age and BMI score at 5 years of age,[58] and protein intake at 2 years of age and BMI at 8 years of age.[82]
- A study conducted with 90 Icelandic infants revealed that the percent of energy from protein intake at 2, 4, 9 and 12 months of age was significantly related to boys' BMI at 6 years of age, while controlling for total energy intake and percent energy from fat and carbohydrates.[83] These relationships were not significant in girls.[83] No statistically significant associations between energy intake and children's BMI were found in these studies.

The Relationship Between Energy Intake and BMI

- A study of 147 Italian children 1 year of age[59] and another study of 70 mid-socioeconomic status white children[81] (2 to 8 years of age from the United States) also found no statistically significant associations between energy intake and BMI at 5 and 8 years of age, respectively.[59,81]

- A 1995 study of a sample of 112 French children reported a statistically significant correlation between BMI at 8 years of age and energy intake at 2 years of age[82]; however, this association disappeared when BMI at 8 years of age or parental BMI were also included in multivariate analyses.
- A longitudinal study of 1379 North Dakota WIC participants 2 to 5 years of age revealed that consumption of high-fat foods, but not the percent of energy from dietary fat, was associated with changes in children's adiposity over a 1-year period.[84] Dietary intake was measured using a semi-quantitative food frequency questionnaire, instead of dietary recalls or records, which were used in most of the other studies. An excess of 1 serving of high-fat food per day was associated with a weight gain of 0.07 kg/year in this regression analysis. One conclusion from this study might be that food intake, rather than macronutrient or estimated energy intake, may be more predictive of young children's weight gain. Differences in dietary collection methods may also account for the differences in the results across studies.

Sweetened Beverages and Obesity

The consumption of sweetened beverages, such as fruit juice, soda and fruit drinks, has been hypothesized to be linked to obesity in young children. Analyses of NHANES III data (1988-1994) revealed a cross-sectional association between reported soda intake and overweight in children 2 to 5 years of age.[85] In another study, 32% of children 2 to 5 years of age recruited from a general pediatrics practice in New York State who consumed more than 12 fluid ounces of juice per day had a BMI above the 90th percentile, while only 9% of children with lower juice intake had BMI above the 90th percentile.[86] In a retrospective study of 10,904 Missouri WIC participants, BMI at 2 to 3 years of age was positively associated with consumption of sweetened beverages, including soda, fruit drinks and other juices, the year prior to BMI measurement.[87]

These results were not replicated in a prospective study of 2- to 5-year-old WIC participants from North Dakota.[88] Separate multivariate analyses examined the association between consumption of fruit juice, fruit drinks, soda and diet soda and change in weight over approximately an 8-month period. The researchers controlled for age, gender, energy intake, change in height and sociodemographic variables in these analyses and found no association between consumption of sweetened beverages and children's BMI.

Furthermore, 2 other longitudinal studies, 1 of US children followed from 2 to 3 years of age[89] and another of German children followed from 3 to 5 years of age,[90] also found no association between fruit juice consumption and BMI.

Evidence supporting the effect of consumption of certain foods or macronutrients on obesity in preschool-aged children is relatively weak and somewhat inconsistent. However, there are data that indicate that low-fat diets can be safely used with young children. Limitations in measuring young children's dietary intakes, because of measurement error and/or biased estimates, complicate attempts to document associations with weight gain and obesity. As a result, clarity may only be possible through experimental studies, such as the Finnish STRIP trial, in which specific foods, macronutrients and/or energy levels are specifically manipulated to examine their effects. As a result, there is an important need to test interventions designed to change potential dietary factors that influence children's weight and to examine the mechanisms that cause young children to gain weight.[4]

Obesity Prevention and Control Interventions for Young Children

To date, only a few behavioral interventions to prevent obesity or CVD risk factors in young children have been described in the research literature.

Healthy Start Program

One such intervention is "Healthy Start," a foodservice program implemented in 6 Head Start programs. Healthy Start significantly reduced the saturated fat content of lunches served in 3 Head Start programs compared to the fat content of lunches in 3 control group sites that did not change the saturated fat content of lunches. After 2 years, the percent of energy from saturated fat consumed by children attending the Healthy Start schools was reduced from 11% at baseline to 8%, while the percent of energy from saturated fat consumed in lunches served at control group programs increased from 10% to 11% during the same time period.[91] In addition, children attending the Healthy Start programs had significantly lower serum cholesterol levels at the end of the 2-year intervention than did the control group children ($P<.001$). However, weight-to-height ratios did not differ between the 2 groups.[92]

Native American Preschool Program

In another trial, a 16-week home-based obesity-prevention program delivered by peer educators to 43 Native American mothers of preschool-aged children resulted in a trend towards lower weight-for-height scores (–.27 ± 1.1 vs +.31 ± 1.1, $P = .06$) and energy intakes for children ($P<.06$), compared to children who received only home-based parenting sessions. These results were not statistically significant.[93] Furthermore, there were no differences between the 2 groups in the proportion of children with a BMI above the 85th or 95th percentiles on the CDC 2000 growth charts or in children's physical activity levels.[93] The obesity-prevention sessions covered topics such as role modeling of healthy eating behavior, food-related parenting and rule setting. Accordingly, mothers in the obesity-prevention group reported decreased "restrictions" based on the subscale from the Child Feeding Questionnaire ($P<.05$).[94] There were no differences in mothers' BMI, dietary intakes or activity levels.

Fit WIC Program

A third study, "Fit WIC," was a feasibility program delivered in a WIC clinic in Virginia. A second WIC clinic served as the (nonrandom) control site. The Fit WIC program encouraged parents of children 2 to 4 years of age to do the following: increase their children's physical activity levels, monitor mealtime behaviors, limit household TV watching, offer water to their children instead of sweetened beverages, encourage household members to consume 5 fruits and vegetables per day, and increase family activities to promote fitness. In addition, WIC staff were asked to model these behaviors. Complementary materials were periodically sent to other community agencies accessed by WIC clientele to further encourage these behaviors. At the end of the 1-year intervention, participants in the Fit WIC program were more likely to report offering water to their children and engaging in active play with them when compared to participants at the comparison site.[95] However, the response rates at posttest were only 65% in the treatment clinic and 43% in the comparison clinic. In addition, the ethnic and racial composition of the clinics differed significantly. The sample from the Fit WIC clinic was 70% Hispanic and 8% black, while the control clinic sample was 37% Hispanic and 23% black.

Hip-Hop to Health Jr.

The most promising preschool intervention to date has been "Hip-Hop to Health Jr.," a 2-year, randomized controlled trial conducted at 12 Head Start sites, involving 420 low-income, predominantly black children.[96] The 14-week obesity-prevention intervention consisted of 20 minutes of healthy eating or exercise lessons and 20 minutes of aerobic activity 3 times a week. The control group received general health education (eg, dental health or safety) once a week for 20 minutes. Weekly parent newsletters and homework assignments were sent home, and parents received a $5 gift certificate for each assignment they completed and returned to the school. Postintervention, there were no differences in BMI between the groups. However, at the 1-year follow-up, the decrease in BMI *z* scores adjusted for age and baseline BMI was significantly greater among children who received the nutrition and exercise curriculum than among children who received the general health curriculum (–0.08 compared to 0.16; $P = .006$). These effects were maintained at the 2-year follow-up, although the difference between groups was not as large. In the nutrition and activity group, BMI *z* scores (adjusted for age and BMI at baseline) had returned to baseline levels, but the adjusted BMI *z* scores of children who received the general health education were, on average, 0.18 standard deviation units higher than their baseline levels ($P<.015$).[96] The differences between the 2 groups were not statistically significant by gender or by level of BMI.

Summary and Conclusions

Childhood obesity has become an important public health problem in the United States and worldwide. Compared to what is known about obesity in older children, adolescents and adults, much less is known about the causes, correlates and consequences of obesity in young children. Young children are generally considered obese if their BMI is at or above the 95th percentile of a reference (eg, the 2000 CDC growth charts or the IOTF BMI references). BMI appears to be the most practical and appropriate measure to define overweight in young children. Based on BMI and related measures, the prevalence of overweight and obesity among young children has been increasing rapidly, mimicking the trends among older children and adolescents. Ethnic/racial differences in the prevalence of overweight among young children also are similar to those seen in older age groups. Increases in the prevalence of overweight and obesity have also been accompanied by increases in the mean levels of BMI in the population.

Although the data are still relatively sparse, BMI and BMI cut-off points in young children modestly predict later adult obesity and are associated with increased CVD risk factors. In fact, some data suggest that elevated BMI in young children is associated with future health risks independent of adult BMI. It is not yet clear whether BMI during early childhood years predicts adult morbidity and mortality. Evidence supporting an effect of the consumption of certain foods or macronutrients on obesity in preschool-aged children is relatively weak and somewhat inconsistent, but there are data to support the safety of low-fat diets in young children.

Unfortunately, a limited amount of data from experimental studies is available to identify the most promising nutrition and/or physical activity strategies for young children. Despite these gaps in our knowledge, however, there appears to be adequate support for testing interventions to prevent and control overweight during young childhood. Existing research has identified a number of potential physiologic, nutritional, behavioral, social, cultural and environmental factors associated with overweight or overweight-promoting eating behaviors in young children. These represent potential targets for obesity prevention and control interventions. However, few attempts have been made to test these factors in experimental trials. The few diet and physical activity interventions tested for young children have demonstrated feasibility and some promise. There is a critical need for additional experimental studies testing a variety of interventions aimed at parents and families, caregivers, educators, health professionals, institutions and policymakers. A "solution-oriented" approach to conducting research is more apt to lead to rapid discovery of innovative and feasible interventions and a better understanding of which moderators and mediators of behavior change will have greater relevance for public health and clinical practice.[97]

References

1. World Health Organization. *Obesity: Preventing and Managing the Global Epidemic: Report of a WHO Consultation on Obesity.* Geneva, Switzerland: World Health Organization; 1998.
2. Kuczmarski R, Ogden C, Grummer-Strawn L, et al. *CDC growth charts: United States.* Hyattsville, Md: National Center for Health Statistics; 2000. Advance data from vital and health statistics; no. 314.
3. Ogden C, Flegal K, Carroll M, Johnson C. Prevalence and trends in overweight among US children and adolescents, 1999-2000. *Journal of the American Medical Association.* 2002;288:1729-1732.
4. National Academy of Sciences, Institute of Medicine, Food and Nutrition Board, Board on Health Promotion and Disease Prevention. *Preventing Childhood Obesity: Health in the Balance.* Washington, DC: The National Academies Press; 2005.

5. Hedley A, Ogden C, Johnson C, Carroll M, Curtin L, Flegal K. Prevalence of overweight and obesity among US children, adolescents, and adults, 1999-2002. *Journal of the American Medical Association.* 2004;291:2847-2850.
6. Flegal K, Troiano RP. Changes in the distribution of body mass index of adults and children in the US population. *International Journal of Obesity.* 2000;24:807-818.
7. Winkleby M, Robinson T, Sundquist J, Kraemer H. Ethnic variation in cardiovascular disease risk factors among children and young adults. *Journal of the American Medical Association.* 1999;281: 1006-1013.
8. Ebbling C, Pawlak D, Ludwig D. Childhood obesity: public-health crisis, common sense cure. *Lancet.* 2002;360:473-482.
9. Dietz W, Robinson TN. Overweight children and adolescents. *New England Journal of Medicine.* 2005;352:2100-2109.
10. Fagot-Campagna A, Saaddine, JB, Flegal K, Engelgau M. Is testing children for type 2 diabetes a lost battle? *Diabetes Care.* 2000;23:1442-1443.
11. Narayan K, Boyle J, Thompson T, Sorensen S, Williamson D. Lifetime risk for diabetes mellitus in the United States. *Journal of the American Medical Association.* 2003;290:1884-1890.
12. Seidel J. Societal and personal costs of obesity. *Experimental Clinical Endocrinology and Diabetes.* 1998;106:7-9.
13. Ulijaszek S, Kerr D. Anthropometric measurement error and the assessment of nutritional status. *British Journal of Nutrition.* 1999;82:165-177.
14. Robinson T. Defining obesity in children and adolescents: clinical approaches. *Critical Review of Food Science and Nutrition.* 1993;33:313-320.
15. Freedman D, Khan L, Serdula M, Srinivasan S, Berenson G. BMI rebound, childhood height, and obesity among adults: the Bogalusa Heart Study. *International Journal of Obesity.* 2001;25:543-549.
16. Freedman D, Khan L, Mei Z, Dietz W, Srinivasan S, Berenson G. Relation of childhood height to obesity among adults: the Bogalusa Heart Study. *Pediatrics.* 2002;109:e23.
17. Bellizzi M, Dietz W. Workshop on childhood obesity: summary of the discussion. *American Journal of Clinical Nutrition.* 1999;70:173S-175S.
18. Cole T, Bellizzi M, Flegal K. Establishing a standard definition for child overweight and obesity worldwide: international survey. *British Medical Journal.* 2000;320:1240-1243.
19. Dietz W, Robinson T. Use of the body mass index (BMI) as a measure of overweight in children and adolescents. *Journal of Pediatrics.* 1998;132:191-193.
20. Himes J. Agreement among anthropometric indicators identifying the fattest adolescents. *International Journal of Obesity.* 1999;23:S18-S21.
21. Himes J, Bouchard C. Validity of anthropometry in classifying youths as obese. *International Journal of Obesity.* 1989;13:183-193.
22. Power C, Lake J, Cole T. Measurement and long-term health risks of child and adolescent fatness. *International Journal of Obesity.* 1997;21:507-526.
23. Troiano R, Flegal K. Overweight children and adolescents: description, epidemiology and demographic. *Pediatrics.* 1998;101:497-504.
24. Ogden C, Kuczmarski R, Flegal K, et al. Centers for Disease Control and Prevention 2000 Growth Charts for the United States: improvements to the 1977 National Center for Health Statistics version. *Pediatrics.* 2002;109:45-60.
25. Flegal K, Ogden C, Wie R, Kuczmarski R, Johnson C. Prevalence of overweight in US children: comparison of US growth charts from the Centers for Disease Control and Prevention with other reference values for body mass index. *American Journal of Clinical Nutrition.* 2001;73:1086-1093.
26. Janssen I, Katzmarzyk P, Srinivasan S, et al. Utility of childhood BMI in the prediction of adulthood disease: comparison of national and international references. *Obesity Research.* 2005;13:1106-1115.
27. Hediger M, Overpeck M, Kuczmarski R, Ruan W. Association between infant breastfeeding and overweight in young children. *Journal of the American Medical Association.* 2001;285:2453-2460.

28. Ogden C, Troiano R, Breifel R, Kuczmarski R, Flegal K, Johnson C. Prevalence of overweight among preschool children in the United States, 1971 through 1994. *Pediatrics.* 1997;99:e1-7.

29. Overpeck M, Hediger M, Ruan W, et al. Stature, weight, and body mass among young US children born at term with appropriate birth weights. *Journal of Pediatrics.* 2000;137:205-213.

30. Jolliffe D. Extent of overweight among US children and adolescents from 1971 to 2000. *International Journal of Obesity.* 2004;28:4-9.

31. Mei Z, Scanlon K, Grummer-Strawn LM, Freedman D, Yip R, Trowbridge F. Increasing prevalence of overweight among US low-income preschool children: the Centers for Disease Control and Prevention Pediatric Nutrition Surveillance, 1983 to 1995. *Pediatrics.* 1998;101:e12.

32. Sherry B, Mei Z, Scanlon K, Mokdad A, Grummer-Strawn LM. Trends in state-specific prevalence of overweight and underweight in 2- through 4-year-old children from low-income families from 1989 through 2000. *Archives of Pediatric and Adolescent Medicine.* 2004;158:1116-1124.

33. Kelsey J, Thompson W, Evans A. *Methods in Observational Epidemiology.* New York, NY: Oxford University Press; 1986.

34. Adams A, Harvey H, Prince R. Association of maternal smoking with overweight at age 3 years in American Indian children. *American Journal of Clinical Nutrition.* 2005;82:393-398.

35. Baruffi G, Hardy C, Waslien C, Uyehara S, Krupitsky D. Ethnic differences in the prevalence of overweight among young children in Hawaii. *Journal of the American Dietetic Association.* 2004;104:1701-1707.

36. Crawford P, Story M, Wang M, Ritchie L, Sabry Z. Ethnic issues in the epidemiology of childhood obesity. *Pediatric Clinics of North America.* 2001;48:855-878.

37. Serdula M, Ivery D, Coates R, Freedman D, Williamson D, Byers T. Do obese children become obese adults? A review of the literature. *Preventive Medicine.* 1993;22:167-177.

38. Asher P. Fat babies and fat children: the prognosis of obesity in the very young. *Archives of Diseases of Children.* 1966;41:672-673.

39. Fisch R, Bilek M, Ulstrom R. Obesity and leanness at birth and their relationship to body habitus in later childhood. *Pediatrics.* 1975;56:521-528.

40. Charney E, Goodman H, McBride M. Childhood antecedents of adult obesity: do chubby infants become obese adults? *New England Journal of Medicine.* 1976;295:6-9.

41. Johnston F, Mack R. Obesity in urban black adolescents of high and low relative weight at 1 year of age. *American Journal of Diseases of Children.* 1978;132:862-864.

42. Zack P, Harlan W, Leaverton P, Cornomi-Huntley J. A longitudinal study of body fatness in childhood and adolescence. *Journal of Pediatrics.* 1979;95:126-130.

43. Stark O, Atkins E, Wolff O, Douglas J. Longitudinal study of obesity in the National Survey of Health and Development. *British Medical Journal.* 1981;283:13-17.

44. Garn S, La Velle M. Two-decade follow-up of fatness in early childhood. *American Journal of Diseases of Children.* 1985;139:181-185.

45. Rolland-Cachera M, Deheeger M, Guilloud-Batouille M, Avons P, Patios E, Sempe M. Tracking the development of adiposity from one month of age to adulthood. *Annals of Human Biology.* 1987;14:219-229.

46. Freedman D, Shear C, Burke G, et al. Persistence of juvenile-onset obesity over eight years: the Bogalusa Heart Study. *American Journal of Public Health.* 1987;77:588-592.

47. Mossberg H. 40-year follow-up of overweight children. *Lancet.* 1989;ii:491-493.

48. Muramatsu S, Sato Y, Miyao M, Muramatsu T, Ito A. A longitudinal study of obesity in Japan: relationship of body habitus between at birth and at age 17. *International Journal of Obesity.* 1990;14:39-45.

49. Prokopec M, Bellisle F. Adiposity in Czech children followed from 1 month of age to adulthood: analysis of individual BMI patterns. *Annals of Human Biology.* 1993;20:517-525.

50. Clarke W, Lauer R. Does childhood obesity track into adulthood? *Critical Review of Food Science and Nutrition.* 1993;33:423-430.

51. Gasser T, Ziegler P, Seifert B, Molinari L, Largo RH, Prader A. Prediction of adult skinfolds and body mass from infancy through adolescence. *Annals of Human Biology.* 1995;22:217-233.

52. Guo S, Wu W, Chumlea W, Roche A. Predicting overweight and obesity in adulthood from body mass index values in childhood and adolescence. *American Journal of Clinical Nutrition.* 2002;76: 653-658.

53. Freedman D, Khan L, Serdula M, Dietz W, Srinivasan S, Berenson G. Racial differences in the tracking of childhood BMI to adulthood. *Obesity Research.* 2005;13:928-935.

54. Freedman D, Khan L, Serdula M, Dietz W, Srinivasan S, Berenson G. The relation of childhood BMI to adult obesity: the Bogalusa Heart Study. *Pediatrics.* 2005;115:22-27.

55. Freedman D, Khan L, Dietz W, Srinivasan S, Berenson G. Relationship of childhood obesity to coronary heart disease risk factors in adulthood: the Bogalusa Heart Study. *Pediatrics.* 2001;108:712-718.

56. Strauss R, Pollack H. Epidemic increase in childhood obesity, 1986-98. *Journal of the American Medical Association.* 2001;286:2845-2848.

57. Whitaker R, Wright J, Pepe M, Seidel K, Dietz W. Predicting obesity in young adulthood from childhood and parental obesity. *New England Journal of Medicine.* 1997;337:869-873.

58. Rolland-Cachera M, Deheeger M, Bellisle F, Sempe M, Guilloud-Batouille M, Patois E. Adiposity rebound in children: a simple indicator for predicting obesity. *American Journal of Clinical Nutrition.* 1984;39:129-135.

59. Scaglioni S, Verduci E, Fiori L, et al. Body mass index rebound and overweight at 8 years of age in hyperphenylalaninaemic children. *Acta Paediatrica.* 2004;93:1596-1600.

60. Siervogel R, Wisemandle W, Maynard L, Guo S, Chumlea W, Towne B. Lifetime overweight status in relation to serial changes in body composition and risk factors for cardiovascular disease: the Fels Longitudinal Study. *Obesity Research.* 2000;8:422-430.

61. Taylor R, Goulding A, Lewis-Barned N, Williams S. Rate of fat gain is faster in girls undergoing early adiposity rebound. *Obesity Research.* 2004;12:1228-1230.

62. Whitaker R, Pepe M, Wright J, Seidel K, Dietz W. Early adiposity rebound and the risk of adult obesity. *Pediatrics.* 1998;101:e5.

63. Wisemandle W, Maynard L, Guo S, Siervogel R. Childhood weight, stature and body mass index among never overweight, early-onset overweight and late-onset overweight groups. *Pediatrics.* 2000;106:e14.

64. Williams S, Davie G, Lam F. Predicting BMI in young adults from childhood data using 2 approaches to modeling adiposity rebound. *International Journal of Obesity.* 1999;23:348-354.

65. Cole T. Children grow and horses race: is the adiposity rebound a critical period for later obesity? *BioMed Central Pediatrics.* 2004;4:6.

66. Dietz W. Adiposity rebound: reality or epiphenomenon? *Lancet.* 2000;356:2027-2028.

67. Freedman D, Dietz W, Tang R, et al. The relation of obesity throughout life to carotid intima-media thickness in adulthood: the Bogalusa Heart Study. *International Journal of Obesity.* 2004;28:159-166.

68. Eriksson J, Forsen T, Tuomilehto J, Osmond C, Barker D. Early growth and coronary heart disease in later life: longitudinal study. *British Medical Journal.* 2001;322:949-953.

69. Adair L, Cole T. Rapid child growth raises blood pressure in adolescent boys who were thin at birth. *Hypertension.* 2003;41:451-456.

70. Law C, Shiell A, Newsome C, et al. Fetal, infant, and childhood growth and adult blood pressure: a longitudinal study from birth to 22 years of age. *Circulation.* 2002;105:1088-1092.

71. Eriksson J, Forsen T, Osmond C, Barker D. Pathways of infant and childhood growth that lead to type 2 diabetes. *Diabetes Care.* 2003;26:3006-3010.

72. Freedman D, Srinivasan S, Cresanta J, Webber L, Berenson G. Serum lipids and lipoproteins. *Pediatrics.* 1987;80(suppl):789-796.

73. Freedman D, Dietz W, Srinivasan S, Berenson G. The relation of overweight to cardiovascular risk factors among children and adolescents: the Bogalusa Heart Study. *Pediatrics.* 1999;103:1175-1182.

74. Berenson G, Srinivasan S, Bao W, Newman W, Tracy R, Wattigney W. Association between multiple cardiovascular risk factors and atherosclerosis in children and young adults. The Bogalusa Heart Study. *New England Journal of Medicine.* 1998;338:1650-1656.
75. Lagstrom H, Jokinen E, Seppanen R. Nutrient intakes by young children in a prospective randomized trial of a low-saturated fat, low-cholesterol diet: the STRIP Baby Project: Special Turku Coronary Risk Factor Intervention Project for Babies. *Archives of Pediatric and Adolescent Medicine.* 1997;151: 181-188.
76. Talvia S, Lagström H, Räsänen M, et al. A randomized intervention since infancy to reduce intake of saturated fat. *Archives of Pediatric and Adolescent Medicine.* 2004;158:41-47.
77. Niinikoski H, Viikari J, Rönnemaa T, et al. Regulation of growth of 7- to 36-month-old children by energy and fat intake in the prospective, randomized STRIP baby trial. *Pediatrics.* 1997;100: 810-816.
78. Shea S, Basch C, Stein A, Contento IR, Irigoyen M, Zybert P. Is there a relationship between dietary fat and stature or growth in children 3 to 5 years of age? *Pediatrics.* 1993;92:579-586.
79. Roger I, Emmet P, Team AS. Fat content of the diet among preschool children in southwest Britain: relationship with growth, blood lipids and iron status. *Pediatrics.* 2001;108:e49.
80. Niinikoski H, Lapinleimu H, Viikari J, et al. Growth until 3 years of age in a prospective, randomized trial of a diet with reduced saturated fat and cholesterol. *Pediatrics.* 1997;99:687-694.
81. Skinner J, Bounds W, Carruth B, Morris M, Ziegler P. Predictors of children's body mass index: a longitudinal study of diet and growth in children aged 2-8 years. *International Journal of Obesity.* 2004;28:476-482.
82. Rolland-Cachera M, Deheeger M, Akrout M, Bellisle F. Influence of macronutrients on adiposity development: a follow up study of nutrition and growth from 10 months to 8 years of age. *International Journal of Obesity and Related Metabolic Disorders.* 1995;19:573-578.
83. Gunnarsdottir I, Thorsdottir I. Relationship between growth and feeding in infancy and body mass index at the age of 6 years. *International Journal of Obesity.* 2003;27:1523-1527.
84. Newby P, Peterson K, Berkey C, Leppert J, Willet W, Colditz G. Dietary composition and weight change among low-income preschool children. *Archives of Pediatric and Adolescent Medicine.* 2003; 157:759-764.
85. Troiano R, Briefel R, Carroll M, Bialostosky K. Energy and fat intakes of children and adolescents in the United States: data from the National Health and Nutrition Examination Surveys. *American Journal of Clinical Nutrition.* 2000;72:1343S-1353S.
86. Dennison B, Rockwell H, Baker S. Excess fruit juice consumption by preschool-aged children is associated with short stature and obesity. *Pediatrics.* 1997;99:15-22.
87. Welsh J, Cogswell M, Rogers S, Rockett H, Mei Z, Grummer-Strawn LM. Overweight among low-income preschool children associated with the consumption of sweet drinks: Missouri, 1999-2002. *Pediatrics.* 2005;115:223-229.
88. Newby P, Peterson K, Berkey C, Leppert J, Willet W, Colditz G. Beverage consumption is not associated with changes in weight and body mass index among low-income preschool children in North Dakota. *Journal of the American Dietetic Association.* 2004;104:1086-1094.
89. Skinner J, Carruth B, Moran J, Houck K, Coletta F. Fruit juice intake is not related to children's growth. *Pediatrics.* 1999;103:58-64.
90. Alexy U, Sichert-Hellert W, Kersting M, Manz F, Schoch G. Fruit juice consumption and the prevalence of obesity and short stature in German preschool children: results of the DONALD Study. Dortmund Nutritional and Anthropometrical Longitudinally Designed. *Journal of Pediatric Gastroenterology and Nutrition.* 1999;29:343-349.
91. Williams C, Bollella M, Strobino B, et al. "Healthy-Start": outcome of an intervention to promote a heart healthy diet in preschool children. *Journal of the American College of Nutrition.* 2002;21:62-71.
92. Williams C, Strobino B, Bollella M, Brotanek J. Cardiovascular risk reduction in preschool children: the "Healthy Start" project. *Journal of the American College of Nutrition.* 2004;23:117-123.

93. Harvey-Berino J, Rourke J. Obesity prevention in preschool Native-American children: a pilot study using home visiting. *Obesity Research.* 2003;11:606-611.

94. Birch L, Fisher J, Castro C, Grimm-Thomas K, Sawyer R, Johnson S. Confirmatory factor analysis of the child feed questionnaire: a measure of parental attitudes, beliefs and practices about child feeding and obesity proneness. *Appetite.* 2001;36:201-210.

95. McGarvey E, Keller A, Forrester M, Williams E, Seward D, Suttle D. Feasibility and benefits of a parent-focused preschool child obesity intervention. *American Journal of Public Health.* 2004;94: 1490-1495.

96. Fitzgibbon ML, Stolley MR, Schiffer L, Van Horn L, KauferChristoffel K, Dyer A. Two-year follow-up results for Hip-Hop to Health Jr.: a randomized controlled trial for overweight prevention in preschool minority children. *Journal of Pediatrics.* 2005;146:618-625.

97. Robinson TN, Sirard JR. Preventing childhood obesity: a solution-oriented research paradigm. *American Journal of Preventive Medicine.* 2005;28:194-201.

Prenatal and Postnatal Flavor Learning in Human Infants

Julie A. Mennella, PhD

Introduction

Flavor preferences are shaped long before infants actually taste their first solid foods. This chapter summarizes the findings from scientific research that reveal that one of the first ways that infants learn about and experience different flavors is through flavor cues in their mothers' amniotic fluid and breast milk. During pregnancy, and later when they are breastfeeding, mothers often include foods in their diets that are specific to their cultures. These foods flavor both the amniotic fluid and breast milk, and thus expose her baby to her food choices. These first taste experiences bias infants' acceptance of particular flavors and may "program" their later food preferences. In this way, culture-specific food preferences are likely initiated very early in life.

Sensory Systems That Detect Flavor

Before pursuing any discussion of early flavor learning, it is necessary to have a basic understanding of taste and smell; the differences between them; and how taste and smell interact to produce the overall impression of flavor. The senses of taste and smell, which are developed in utero but continue to mature postnatally,[1] serve as gatekeepers, determining which foods gain admission to the digestive tract. Taste and smell evolved to help humans reject foods that are harmful and to seek out foods that are beneficial and pleasurable.[2] For example, it has been suggested that the heightened preference for sweet tastes among infants and children, which is evident around the world, evolved to attract them to sources of high energy during periods of maximal growth.[3-6] The rejection of bitter tastes evolved, in part, to protect children from ingesting poisons.[7]

The receptors for taste stimuli — which are located on the tongue and other parts of the oral cavity — and the receptors for olfactory stimuli — which are located high in the nasal chambers — probe the environment and convert the chemicals that are detected into specific patterns of neuronal activity. When foods or liquids are taken into the mouth, the perceptions that arise through the senses of taste and smell combine to determine flavor. However, these perceptions are often confused and misappropriated.[8] For example, the sensations produced by vanilla, fish, chocolate and coffee are often erroneously attributed to the taste system per se. In fact, there are only a small number of primary taste qualities (eg, sweet, salty, bitter, sour and savory tastes) that can be perceived by all areas of the tongue. Smell sensations, on the other hand, encompass thousands of diverse qualities. The receptors for the olfactory system are stimulated during inhalation (the orthonasal route) and also during sucking in infants and during deglutition in both children and adults when molecules reach the receptors by passing from the oral cavity through the nasal pharynx (the retronasal route). It is the retronasal stimulation arising from the molecules of foods that produces the predominant flavor sensations we experience.

Amniotic Fluid and Breast Milk Reflect the Mother's Culture

A fundamental feature of mammals is that their first foods — amniotic fluid and mother's milk — are flavored by the foods eaten by the mother during pregnancy and lactation, respectively. Research on a variety of nonhuman mammalian species revealed that young animals develop preferences for flavors experienced in amniotic fluid and their mothers' milk which, in turn, facilitate the transition to solid foods.[9-11] For example, the growth rate of weanling pigs improved when a flavor included in the sow's feed during lactation was added to the weanling's feed.[12] In addition, weanling animals actively seek and prefer the flavors of the foods eaten by their mother during nursing, and are more likely to accept unfamiliar flavors if they experience a variety of different flavors during the nursing period.[13]

Because this learning occurs when flavors are experienced during either gestation or lactation,[10] it has been hypothesized that such redundancy of dietary information may be important biologically. It provides complementary routes of transferring information regarding the types of foods available in the environment, should the mother's diet change during the course of pregnancy or lactation.[10]

At weaning, a young animal must learn what to eat and how to forage. Exposure to a variety of dietary flavors in amniotic fluid and mother's milk may be one of several ways that the mother teaches her young what foods are "safe."[14] Research indicates that young animals tend to prefer a diet similar to that of their mothers.[9,11,12,15]

During the past 15 years, researchers have expanded upon the findings in nonhuman animals, examining feeding and eating in the human mother-infant dyad. These studies have revealed that one source of chemosensory stimulation for the fetus is the maternal diet.[16-18] That is, the environment in which the fetus lives, the amniotic sac, changes as a function of the food choices the mother makes. The flavors of the mother's diet are transmitted to and flavor the amniotic fluid. The specific flavors that the fetus experiences in the amniotic fluid lead to an increased enjoyment of and preference for these flavors at birth and later during weaning. For example, exposure to the flavors of garlic or anise in utero resulted in less aversive facial displays and increased mouthing and orienting during exposure to those odors during the immediate postpartum period.[17,18]

Infants subsequently experience some of these same flavors in their mother's milk, which is a predominantly sweet liquid. Like amniotic fluid, human milk is flavored by the foods, spices and beverages that mothers ingest or inhale (eg, tobacco).[19-23] Because amniotic fluid and breast milk share a commonality in their flavor profiles that reflects the foods eaten by the mother, breast milk may actually act as a "bridge" between the early in utero flavor experiences and the later flavor experiences of the infant's solid-food diet.

The sweetness and the textural properties of human milk, such as its viscosity and the degree to which it coats the infant's mouth, vary from mother to mother.[24] Therefore, breastfeeding, unlike formula feeding, provides the infant with the potential for a rich variety of chemosensory experiences. The types and intensity of flavors experienced in breast milk are different for each child and uniquely identify the culture into which she or he is born.

Examining Prenatal and Postnatal Flavor Learning

My colleagues and I conducted an experiment to test the hypothesis that pre- and postnatal flavor experiences enhance the acceptance and enjoyment of flavors during infancy. We randomly assigned 46 pregnant women who planned on breastfeeding their infants to 1 of 3 groups[25]:

- A group that drank carrot juice for several days per week during the last trimester of pregnancy (but drank water and refrained from eating carrots or drinking carrot juice during lactation)
- A group that drank water and refrained from eating carrots or drinking carrot juice during the last trimester of pregnancy but drank carrot juice for a similar time period during lactation
- A control group that drank water and refrained from drinking carrot juice and eating carrot during both pregnancy and lactation

Approximately 4 weeks after the mothers began adding cereal to their infants' diet, and before the infants had ever been fed foods or juices containing the flavor of carrots, the infants were videotaped as they were fed cereal. During 1 test session, the mothers fed the infants cereal prepared with water; during the other test session they fed them cereal prepared with carrot juice.

Similar to the kinds of reactions observed in other young mammals,[9,10,15] the infants who had been exposed to the flavor of carrots in either amniotic fluid or their mothers' milk reacted differently to that flavor in a solid food than did the control group infants who had not been exposed previously to the flavor of carrots. Specifically, infants who had been exposed to the flavor of carrots displayed fewer negative facial expressions while eating the carrot-flavored cereal than they did when eating the plain cereal. Moreover, the mothers of those infants who were exposed to carrots prenatally perceived that their infants enjoyed the carrot-flavored cereal more than they did the plain cereal. Postnatal exposure to carrot flavor through mother's milk resulted in similar responses in infants, thus highlighting the importance of a varied diet for both pregnant and lactating women.

A recent study of women living in several regions of Mexico[26] found that despite regional differences in cuisine, there were striking similarities in the types of foods eaten by mothers during pregnancy and fed to infants during weaning. Mothers reported that they ate more fruits and vegetables during pregnancy and lactation because they preferred their taste, craved them or because they were advised to do so by their mothers, physicians or both. The first food these mothers fed their infants was a fruit or a vegetable. Thus, the foods eaten by the mothers became the basis of the infants' diets during weaning. The types and intensity of flavors experienced in utero and in mothers' milk may identify the flavor principles of the culture to which infants belong, as well as enhance acceptance of culture-specific foods during weaning.

Flavor Acceptance Is Also Linked to Diet Variety

Infants' acceptance of a flavor may not require that they experience that flavor per se in utero or during lactation. Rather, for both human infants[27] and young animals,[13] experience with a variety of flavors in utero and during lactation increases the likelihood that they will accept a variety of novel foods during weaning. Breastfed infants were more willing to accept a novel vegetable when it was first fed to them than were formula-fed infants.[28] One explanation for this behavior is that, unlike the formula-fed infant who experiences a monotony of flavors in infant formula, the breastfed infant is exposed to many different flavors in breast milk, establishing early the pattern of a diversified diet.

To test this hypothesis, my colleagues and I conducted an experimental study[27] where we evaluated acceptance of a novel vegetable (ie, pureed carrot) and a novel meat (ie, pureed chicken) before and after a 9-day exposure period in infants. We randomly assigned infants to 1 of 3 groups:

- A group who was fed carrots each day during a 9-day period
- A group who was fed potato each day during a 9-day period
- A group who was fed a variety of vegetables that differed in taste, smell and texture during a 9-day period

We found that the infants repeatedly fed carrots and infants who were fed a variety of vegetables — but not those infants fed potatoes — ate significantly more of the carrots after the exposure period. Infants who ate a variety of vegetables also ingested more of a novel food (chicken) than did those infants who were repeatedly fed carrots or potatoes. These findings were the first experimental evidence to demonstrate that exposure to flavor variety enhances acceptance of novel foods in human infants.[27]

Learning About Flavors in Formula

Although the early flavor experiences of infants who are formula fed are less varied than are the flavor experiences of breastfed infants, formula-fed infants can detect flavors in their formulas and they develop preferences for their own formula's specific flavor profile.[23,29,30] Infants' responses to protein hydrolysate formulas such as Nutramigen™ and Alimentum™ provide a clear example of this. These formulas, which were designed to supply infants with protein nutrients in a "predigested" form as amino acids and small peptides — to lessen the burden of digestion and to prevent allergenicity — are extremely unpalatable to adults and older children. Their unpalatability is likely the result of the formula processing and composition, because many amino acids and small peptides taste sour and bitter — and are characterized by unpleasant volatiles. Modified hydrolysate formulas (in which 1 or several amino acids are deleted or reduced) also are fed to infants who suffer from certain genetic metabolism disorders (eg, phenylketonuria or PKU, or maple syrup urine disease).

Over the past decade, this class of hydrolyzed protein-based infant formulas has served as a model system for the study of early flavor programming. Using 1 of these formulas, Nutramigen, my colleagues and I found that early exposure to Nutramigen resulted in a complete shift in acceptance of its flavor by infants — from absolute dislike at first try to eager acceptance after multiple feedings.[29-33] Because the 2 most popular brands of hydrolysate formulas sold in the United States, Nutramigen and Alimentum, each have distinctive flavors, we subsequently sought to determine whether infants fed Nutramigen would learn to prefer its familiar flavor over the unfamiliar flavor of Alimentum and vice versa. The research showed us that this was clearly the case. The preference pattern that developed in infants was specific to the flavor profile they experienced. Whether this shift in hedonic tone depends on developmental and experiential changes in response to the formula's volatile components (olfactory imprinting) or its taste (taste imprinting), or both, remains to be determined.

The Effects of Early Flavor Learning Continue Into Childhood

Experimental research also suggests that the effects of early exposure linger into childhood. Children who were fed hydrolysate formulas during infancy had heightened preferences for sour tastes, as well as for the aroma and taste of their specific formula, even several years after the last exposure to the formula.[34,35] Clinical observations of children with PKU (who are fed a type of hydrolysate formula) suggest that the effects of early exposure continue even into adolescence. Adolescent children with PKU who discontinued using their modified hydrolysate formula could, albeit with some difficulty, return to using the formulas they were reared on as infants.[36] When these formulas were reintroduced during adolescence to test the feasibility of returning older children with classical phenylketonuria (PKU) to therapeutically and nutritionally adequate phenylalanine-restricted diets after 8 to 13 years of unrestricted diets, the adolescents accepted them relatively well and reported that their most-preferred flavors, which they often added to the formulas, included lemon (ie, sour) and carbonated beverages.[37] In addition, another study showed that children and adolescents with PKU preferred their "bad-tasting" formula to the taste of a new formulation that was more palatable to children and adults not previously exposed to the modified hydrolysate formulas.[38]

Because these formulas are extremely unpalatable to adolescents who have not had previous exposure to them as infants, this *relative* ease of return by adolescents previously exposed to the modified hydrolysate formula could be a function of the long-term effects of their prior flavor experience. As we observed in our studies of infants,[30] the characteristic flavor of the formula experienced in early life is "programmed" and remains preferred for a considerable time thereafter.

Why is there a time period in early infancy important for the acceptance of hydrolyzed formulas? Presuming that the acceptance is an adaptive reason, it has less to do with these hydrolyzed protein formulas themselves than with early flavor learning itself. Indeed, these observations with formulas point to a fundamental aspect of early flavor learning: When an infant is exposed to a particular flavor in amniotic fluid or breast milk — even a relatively unpalatable flavor — and is exposed again to that flavor later on in life, he or she accepts that flavor more readily than does a child without such flavor experience as an infant. Presumably, learning (eg, elimination of neophobia, conditioning or "mere exposure") has occurred.

Teleologically, one can argue that the infant has acquired information that the food associated with the flavor is not dangerous or is nutritionally valuable, or both. It is important for the infant to accept, and be particularly attracted to, the flavors consumed by the mother. These are the flavors that are associated with nutritious foods, or at least, the foods the infant has access to, and hence the foods to which the infant will be exposed the earliest. Prenatal and early postnatal exposures to flavors predispose the infant to favorably respond to the now-familiar flavor, which, in turn, facilitates the transition from fetal life through the breastfeeding period to the initiation of a varied solid-food diet.

Long-Term Benefits of Breastfeeding

The long-term consequences of early milk feedings on the development of food and flavor preferences have been the subject of a few studies in recent years. In an 8-year longitudinal study conducted in the United States, it was determined that fruit and vegetable consumption by school-aged children was predicted by breastfeeding duration, by food-related experiences during early life, or by mothers' preferences.[39,40] For example, consumption of a variety of vegetables by school-aged children was predicted by mothers' vegetable preferences, whereas consumption of a variety of fruits by school-aged children was predicted by breast-feeding duration and early experience with either fruit variety or fruit exposure. The strongest predictors of the number of foods liked by children at 8 years of age were the number of foods they liked at 4 years of age and their food neophobia scores. Mothers' and children's food preferences were significantly but moderately related. Foods that were disliked by mothers typically were not offered to children. Similar findings have been reported in the United Kingdom[41] and France.[42] Clearly, more research in this area is needed. However, the finding that infants learn through flavor cues in breast milk suggests 1 mechanism (but not the only one) underlying these associations.

References

1. Mennella JA. Taste and smell. In: Swaiman KF, Ashwall S, eds. *Pediatric Neurology: Principles and Practice.* 3rd ed. Philadelphia, Pa: CV Mosby Company; 1999;104-113.
2. Cowart BJ. Taste, our body's gustatory gatekeeper. *Cerebrum.* 2005;7:7-22.
3. Beauchamp GK. Factors affecting sweetness. In: Corti A, ed. *Low-Calorie Sweeteners: Present and Future.* Basel, Switzerland: Karger; 1999:10-17.

4. Simmen B, Hladik CM. Sweet and bitter taste discrimination in primates: scaling effects across species. *Folia Primatologica (Basel).* 1998;69:129-138.
5. Drewnowski A. Sensory control of energy density at different life stages. *Proceedings of the Nutrition Society.* 2000;59:239-244.
6. Coldwell SE, Oswald TK. Growth-rate differs between children with adult-like versus child-like sugar preference. *Journal of Dental Research.* 2004;83(special issue A):Abstract 0740.
7. Glendinning JI. Is the bitter rejection response always adaptive? *Physiology and Behavior.* 1994;56:1217-1227.
8. Rozin P. "Taste-smell confusions" and the duality of the olfactory sense. *Perception and Pyschophysics.* 1982;31:397-401.
9. Galef BG, Clark MM. Mother's milk and adult presence: two factors determining initial dietary selection by weanling rats. *Journal of Comparative Physiology and Psychology.* 1972;8:220-225.
10. Bilko A, Altbacker V, Hudson R. Transmission of food preference in the rabbit: the means of information transfer. *Physiology and Behavior.* 1994;56:907-912.
11. Early DM, Provenza FD. Food flavor and nutritional characteristics alter dynamics of food preference in lambs. *Journal of Animal Sciences.* 1998;76:728-734.
12. Campbell RG. A note on the use of feed flavor to stimulate the feed intake of weaning pigs. *Animal Production.* 1976;23:417-419.
13. Capretta PJ, Petersik JT, Steward DJ. Acceptance of novel flavors is increased after early experience of diverse taste. *Nature.* 1975;254:689-691.
14. Rozin P. The selection of food by rats, humans and other animals. In: Rosenblatt J, Hinde RA, Beer C, Shaw E, eds. *Advances in the Study of Behaviors.* New York, NY: Academic Press; 1976:21-76.
15. Nolte DL, Provenza FD, Balph DF. The establishment and persistence of food preferences in lambs exposed to selected foods. *Journal of Animal Sciences.* 1990;68:998-1002.
16. Mennella JA, Johnson A, Beauchamp GK. Garlic ingestion by pregnant women alters the odor of amniotic fluid. *Chemical Senses.* 1995;20:207-209.
17. Hepper PG. Adaptive fetal learning: prenatal exposure to garlic affects postnatal preferences. *Animal Behavior.* 1988;36:935-936.
18. Schaal B, Marlier L, Soussignan R. Human fetuses learn odors from their pregnant mother's diet. *Chemical Senses.* 2000;25:729-737.
19. Mennella JA, Beauchamp GK. Smoking and the flavor of breast milk. *New England Journal of Medicine.* 1998;339:1559-1560.
20. Mennella JA, Beauchamp GK. Beer, breast feeding, and folklore. *Developmental Psychobiology.* 1993;26:459-466.
21. Mennella JA, Beauchamp GK. The transfer of alcohol to human milk: effects on flavor and the infant's behavior. *New England Journal of Medicine.* 1991;325:981-985.
22. Mennella JA, Beauchamp GK. Maternal diet alters the sensory qualities of human milk and the nursling's behavior. *Pediatrics.* 1991;88:737-744.
23. Mennella JA, Beauchamp GK. The human infants' responses to vanilla flavors in human milk and formula. *Infant Behavior and Development.* 1995;19:13-19.
24. Barker E. *Sensory Evaluation of Human Milk* [master's thesis]. Winnipeg, Canada: University of Manitoba; 1980.
25. Mennella JA, Jagnow CP, Beauchamp GK. Prenatal and postnatal flavor learning by human infants. *Pediatrics.* 2001;107:E88
26. Mennella JA, Turnbull B, Ziegler PJ, Martinez H. Infant feeding practices and early flavor experiences in Mexican infants: an intra-cultural study. *Journal of the American Dietetic Association.* 2005;105:908-915.
27. Gerrish CJ, Mennella JA. Flavor variety enhances food acceptance in formula-fed infants. *American Journal of Clinical Nutrition.* 2001;73:1080-1085.
28. Sullivan S, Birch LL. Infant dietary experience and acceptance of solid foods. *Pediatrics.* 1994;93: 271-277.

29. Mennella JA, Beauchamp GK. Understanding the origin of flavor preferences. *Chemical Senses.* 2005;30 (suppl 1):i242-i243.
30. Mennella JA, Griffin CE, Beauchamp GK. Flavor programming during infancy. *Pediatrics.* 2004; 113:840-845.
31. Mennella JA, Beauchamp GK. Developmental changes in the acceptance of protein hydrolysate formula. *Journal of Developmental and Behavioral Pediatrics.* 1996;17:386-391.
32. Mennella JA, Beauchamp GK. Exploring the beginning of flavor preferences. *Chemical Senses.* 2005;30:242-243.
33. Mennella JA, Beauchamp GK. Development and bad taste. *Pediatric Allergy, Asthma and Immunology.* 1998;12:161-163.
34. Liem DG, Mennella JA. Sweet and sour preferences during childhood: role of early experiences. *Developmental Psychobiology.* 2002;41:388-395.
35. Mennella JA, Beauchamp GK. Flavor experiences during formula feeding are related to preferences during childhood. *Early Human Development.* 2002;68:71-82.
36. Schuett VE, Brown ES, Michals K. Reinstitution of diet therapy in PKU patients from 22 clinics. *American Journal of Public Health.* 1985;75:39-42.
37. Hogan SE, Gates RD, MacDonald GW, Clarke JT. Experience with adolescents with phenylketonuria returned to phenylalanine-restricted diets. *Journal of the American Dietetic Association.* 1986;86:1203-1207.
38. Owada M, Aoki K, Kitagawa T. Taste preferences and feeding behaviour in children with phenylketonuria on a semisynthetic diet. *European Journal of Pediatrics.* 2000;159:846-850.
39. Skinner JD, Carruth BR, Bounds W, Ziegler P, Reidy K. Do food-related experiences in the first 2 years of life predict dietary variety in school-aged children? *Journal of Nutrition and Educational Behavior.* 2002;34:310-315.
40. Skinner JD, Carruth BR, Wendy B, Ziegler PJ. Children's food preferences: a longitudinal analysis. *Journal of the American Dietetic Association.* 2002;102:1638-1646.
41. Cooke LJ, Wardle J, Gibson EL, Sapochnik M, Sheilham A, Lawson M. Demographic, familial and trait predictors of fruit and vegetable consumption by preschool children. *Public Health Nutrition.* 2004;7:295-302.
42. Nicklaus, S, Boggio V, Chabanet C, Issanchou S. A prospective study of food preferences in children. *Appetite.* 2004;15:805-818.

Breastfeeding and Other Infant Feeding Practices That May Influence Child Obesity

Kathryn G. Dewey, PhD

Introduction

During the past 6 years, a wealth of new studies on the relationship between breastfeeding and child obesity has sparked intense interest in this issue, particularly given the continuing trend towards higher rates of child obesity in the United States[1] and elsewhere.[2] The effect of other infant feeding practices on obesity, such as bottle-feeding behaviors, early introduction of solid foods and provision of large amounts of juice or sweetened beverages, is also of great interest, although there is less evidence on these relationships.

This chapter is organized into the following 5 sections:

- Growth patterns during infancy
- The association between breastfeeding and overweight in childhood and adolescence
- Potential explanations for the association between breastfeeding and lower risk of child overweight
- Other infant feeding behaviors that may influence the risk of child obesity
- Clinical and public health implications and intervention strategies

Growth Patterns During Infancy

Various infant feeding practices are associated with weight differences during infancy. For example, the DARLING study[3] documented differences in growth from birth to 2 years of age between cohorts of breastfed and formula-fed infants that were matched for characteristics such as parental socioeconomic status, education, weight status and infant birth weight. In the breastfed group, infants were exclusively breastfed until at least 4 months of age and continued to receive breast milk as their sole source of milk until at least 12 months of age. The formula-fed group of infants was fed cow's milk formula as the predominant or sole source of milk starting at birth or within the first few weeks, and continuing until at least 12 months of age. Both groups of infants increased in body fatness during the first 6 months, but became leaner thereafter, with fatness decreasing more sharply in the breastfed group than in the formula-fed group. There were significant differences between the 2 groups in the sum of skinfolds (at 5 sites) between 9 and 17 months of age and in estimated body fat percentage between 5 and 24 months of age.

In a subsequent analysis of 7 studies in North America and northern Europe that documented growth of infants who were breastfed for at least 12 months (1 of which was the DARLING study), similar results were found.[4] In all 7 studies, the mean weight-for-length *z* score between 3 and 12 months of age showed a declining trend, suggesting that the breastfed cohorts were leaner than the National Center for Health Statistics (NCHS) reference population (which was based on mostly bottle-fed infants). The mean weight-for-length of the breastfed infants at 12 months of age was about 0.2 to 0.6 standard deviations (SDs) below the NCHS median. Results of other studies generally confirm that a longer duration of breastfeeding is associated with lower weight-for-length or body mass index (BMI, which is weight/height, measured by kg/m^2) in later infancy.[5-8]

The Association Between Breastfeeding and Overweight in Childhood and Adolescence

A key question is whether overweight during childhood, not just during infancy, is associated with breastfeeding and duration of breastfeeding. In this overview, only studies that met the following 3 criteria were included:

- **A sample size of at least 100 infants per feeding group.** When examining obesity as an outcome, sample sizes of at least 100 infants are needed to obtain a valid prevalence estimate.
- **Age at follow-up > 3 years.** This criterion was imposed in order to examine obesity during childhood and adolescence, rather than only the lingering effects of possible differences by feeding mode that occur during infancy.
- **Outcomes that include the percentage of children who were overweight or obese, not just the mean weight-for-length or BMI.** This criterion was included in order to focus on the right-hand tail of the distribution. There is evidence that breastfeeding reduces the extremes at both ends — both overweight and underweight[9] — which would result in a reduced prevalence of obesity but no difference in mean BMI.

Table 1 shows the 21 studies that met these 3 criteria. Six studies focused primarily on children ≤ 5 years of age (preschool-aged children), 8 studies examined mostly school-aged children and 7 studies focused on adolescents or included children representing a wide age range. The studies varied in sample size, definition of feeding groups and the definition of overweight or obesity. One key methodologic feature was the ability to control for the potentially confounding influence of parental overweight. In most industrialized countries, breastfeeding is less common among overweight mothers than it is among mothers of normal weight. This is partly because of socioeconomic differences, but it may also have biologic origins because obesity is thought to impair the establishment of lactation.[10] Because child obesity is strongly linked to parental obesity (for both genetic and environmental reasons), it is important to control for the latter when examining the association between breastfeeding and child obesity. In the results column of Table 1, the 16 studies that included maternal BMI as a covariate in the analyses are noted.

Table 1. Studies Examining the Relationship Between Feeding Mode During Infancy and Obesity in Childhood and Adolescence

Studies of Preschool-Aged Children

Author Year, Site	N	Age, y	Feeding Groups*	Outcome Measures**	Results[†]
Armstrong et al 2002, Scotland	32,200	3-4	EBF vs EFF at 6-8 wk	BMI > 95th BMI > 98th	AOR 0.72[‡] AOR 0.70[‡]
Bogen et al 2004, USA	73,458	4	BF < 8 wk, 8-15 wk, 16-26 wk, > 26 wk (+/- concurrent FF)	BMI ≥ 95th	AOR 0.71[‡] for 16-26 wk w/o FF[§]
Hediger et al 2001, USA	2685	3-5	Ever BF vs EFF, Duration full BF	BMI 85-95th BMI ≥ 95th	AOR 0.63[‡§] AOR 0.84[§]
Grummer-Strawn and Mei 2004, USA	177,304	4	BF < 1, 1-3, 3-6, 6-12 or ≥ 12 mo, vs EFF	BMI ≥ 95th	AOR for white, non-Hispanic[§] 0.70[‡] (BF 6-12 mo) 0.49[‡] (BF ≥ 12 mo)
O'Callaghan et al 1997, Australia	4062	5	BF duration	BMI 85-95th BMI > 95th	NS[§] NS[§]
Burke et al 2005, Australia	2087	1-8	EFF vs BF ≤ 4 mo, 5-8 mo, 9-12 mo, > 12 mo	BMI ≥ 95th	Highest risk[‡] in BF ≤ 4 mo group[§]
Studies of School-Aged Children					
Von Kries et al 1999, Germany	9357	5-6	Ever BF vs EFF, Duration EBF	BMI > 90th BMI > 97th	AOR 0.79[‡] AOR 0.75[‡]
Bergmann et al 2003, Germany	480	6	BF ≥ or < 3 mo	BMI > 90th BMI > 97th	AOR 0.53[‡§] AOR 0.46[‡§]
Liese et al 2001, Germany	2108	9-10	Ever BF vs EFF, Duration BF or EBF	BMI > 90th	AOR 0.66[‡]
Li et al 2005, USA	2636	2-14	BF 1-3 mo, ≥ 4 mo, vs EFF	BMI ≥ 95th	AOR 0.60 for BF ≥ 4 mo[§]
Reilly et al 2005, UK	8234	7	EBF ≥ 2 mo or < 2 mo, vs EFF	BMI ≥ 95th	Lower risk[‡] if EBF, only if mother nonsmoking[§]
Toschke et al 2002, Czech Republic	33,768	6-14	Ever BF vs EFF, Duration BF	BMI > 90th BMI > 97th	AOR 0.80[‡§] AOR 0.80[‡§]
Gillman et al 2001, USA	15,341	9-14	Predominantly BF vs Predominantly FF from 0-6 mo	BMI > 95th	AOR 0.78[‡§]
Wadsworth et al 1999, UK	3731	6	Ever BF vs EFF, Duration BF	BMI > 90th BMI > 97th	RR 0.95 RR 0.88

*EBF = exclusively breastfed, EFF = exclusively formula fed, BF = breastfed, FF = formula fed

**BMI = body mass index, percentile for age

[†]AOR = adjusted odds ratio, NS = not significant, RR = relative risk

[‡]$P<.05$

[§]Covariates include maternal BMI

Table 1. Studies Examining the Relationship Between Feeding Mode During Infancy and Obesity in Childhood and Adolescence (continued)

Studies of Adolescents

Author Year, Site	N	Age, y	Feeding Groups*	Outcome Measures**	Results†
Kvaavik et al 2005, Norway	635	11-16	BF > 3 mo vs EFF	BMI > 95th	AOR 0.15‡§
Kramer 1981, Canada	427	12-18	Ever BF vs EFF, Duration full BF	>120% median wt for ht	RR 0.31‡§
Tulldahl et al 1999, Sweden	781	17-18	EBF > 2 mo vs EBF ≤ 2 mo	BMI > 85th	RR 0.70‡
Poulton et al 2001, New Zealand	1037	3-26	BF > 6 mo vs EFF	BMI > 25	AOR 0.25-1.01§
Li et al 2003, UK	2631	4-18	Duration BF vs BF < 1 wk	BMI > 95th	NS§
Victora et al 2003, Brazil	2250	18 (male)	Duration predominant BF	BMI > 85th Skinfolds > 90th	Significant linear trend§
Nelson et al 2005, USA	11,998 850 sib pairs	12-21	BF ≥ 9 mo vs EFF	BMI ≥ 85th	AOR 0.78‡ (F)§ AOR 0.83 (M) NS for sib pairs

*EBF = exclusively breastfed, EFF = exclusively formula fed, BF = breastfed, FF = formula fed
**BMI = body mass index, percentile for age
†AOR = adjusted odds ratio, NS = not significant, RR = relative risk
‡$P<.05$
§Covariates include maternal BMI

Results for Preschool-Aged Children

Among the 6 studies on preschool-aged children, 5 showed a relationship between breastfeeding and reduced risk of overweight or obesity, at least for certain subgroups:

- The study by Armstrong et al[11] evaluated obesity among 32,200 preschool-aged children in Scotland. The investigators compared the prevalence of obesity between groups who had been either exclusively breastfed or exclusively formula-fed during the first 6 to 8 weeks of life. For both outcomes assessed (BMI > 95th, BMI > 98th percentile), the adjusted odds ratio (AOR) was significant, showing a lower risk of obesity in the breastfed group after controlling for socioeconomic status, birth weight and gender.

- Bogen and colleagues[12] examined overweight (BMI > 95th percentile) at 4 years of age among 73,458 low-income children in the United States. Feeding groups were based on breastfeeding duration and age of formula initiation. After controlling for several potential confounding factors, breastfeeding was associated with a reduced risk of overweight, but only among white infants whose mothers did not smoke during pregnancy. In this subgroup, the lowest AOR (0.55, relative to never breastfed) was for the group breastfed > 26 weeks, without concurrent formula use.
- The study by Hediger et al[13] used data from the US NHANES III survey for 2685 children 3 to 5 years of age. The investigators defined the feeding groups as ever breastfed or exclusively formula-fed, as well as by the duration of full breastfeeding (no liquids other than breast milk or water). There were 2 outcomes in the analyses: overweight but not obese (85th-94th percentile) and obese (> 95th percentile). Among children who were ever breastfed, breastfeeding was not significantly associated with obesity, but was predictive of a lower risk of overweight (and of the combined categories of overweight and obese, ie, > 85th percentile) (Hediger, personal communication). Hediger and colleagues were able to control for maternal BMI, as well as the child's birth weight, race/ethnicity, gender, age and the timing of introduction of solid foods.
- The study by Grummer-Strawn and Mei[9] had the largest sample size: 177,304 children in the United States at 4 years of age (although data on maternal characteristics such as BMI were available for only 12,587 children in the sample). The researchers found a dose-response relationship between the duration of breastfeeding and a lower risk of overweight among non-Hispanic white children, but no significant association among Hispanics or non-Hispanic black children. Among non-Hispanic whites, the AOR for breastfeeding > 12 months of age (versus never breastfeeding) was 0.49.
- O'Callaghan et al[14] studied 4062 children 5 years of age in Australia. After controlling for birth weight, gender, gestational age, infant feeding problems, infant sleeping problems, parental BMI, education and income, the investigators found no significant association between duration of breastfeeding and overweight or obesity. The data were analyzed using 6 categories for the duration of breastfeeding, but when recategorized into 2 groups, inspection of their data indicated that the prevalence of obesity was 4.1% (67/1652) among children breastfed for at least 4 months compared to 5.5% (124/2257) among those breastfed for less than 4 months

(relative risk = 0.75). This difference did not appear to be greatly altered after adjustment for confounding factors, and is of similar magnitude to the significant effects observed in several other studies in Table 1.

- Burke and colleagues[6] evaluated obesity among 2087 children 1 to 8 years of age in Australia. When compared to children breastfed for > 12 months of age, children breastfed for ≤ 4 months (AOR 1.87) had a significantly higher risk for obesity, but those children who were never breastfed (AOR 1.02) did not. However, only 12% of children in the study were never breastfed, and although they did not differ in birth weight or gestational age from those who were breastfed, it is possible that they had characteristics that led to not being breastfed (eg, poorer health status) and also limited subsequent weight gain. This potential for reverse causation raises the possibility that the results of studies may differ in populations with low (vs high) rates of initiation of breastfeeding. In a country like Australia, where initiation rates are high, nonbreastfed children are more likely to be a "biased" group than in countries where initiation rates are lower.

Results for School-Aged Children

Among the 8 studies primarily focused on school-aged children, all but 1 showed an association between breastfeeding and lower risk of overweight:

- The 3 studies conducted in Germany[15-17] all reported lower rates of overweight among children who had been breastfed, but only the study by Bergmann et al[15] included maternal overweight as a covariate. This study followed children longitudinally from birth to 6 years of age. The formula-fed children were more likely to be overweight as infants (19% compared to 10% in the breastfed cohort). The difference between feeding groups subsequently became insignificant at 1 to 4 years of age, but reemerged at 5 to 6 years of age. At 6 years of age, the percentage overweight was nearly 30% in the formula-fed group, compared to 12% in the breastfed group. These results indicate that the breastfeeding "effect," if it is indeed causal, is expressed most strongly after 4 years of age.
- Of the other 5 studies in this age group,[18-22] 4 included maternal overweight as a covariate:
  - Li et al[18] examined overweight in 2636 children in the United States between 2 and 14 years of age. The AOR for overweight in children who had been breastfed for ≥ 4 months was 0.6 (P = .06 for linear

trend), controlling for numerous covariates. There was an additive interaction between maternal obesity prior to pregnancy and lack of breastfeeding: Overweight occurred in 31.5% of children who were never breastfed and were born to obese mothers, compared to 6.0% of children who were breastfed for ≥ 4 months and were born to mothers with a BMI < 25.

- Reilly et al[19] evaluated early life risk factors for obesity in 8234 children in the United Kingdom who were 7 years of age at the time of measurement. Breastfeeding was associated with reduced risk of obesity among children of nonsmoking mothers, but not associated with reduced risk of obesity among children of mothers who smoked during pregnancy.
- Toschke and colleagues[20] evaluated the weight status of 33,768 children 6 to 14 years of age in the Czech Republic. After controlling for parental BMI, education level, maternal smoking, child birth weight, time spent watching television, number of siblings, physical activity levels and dietary factors, breastfeeding was associated with a reduced risk of both overweight and obesity.
- Gillman et al[21] studied the risk of obesity in more than 15,000 children in the United States who had been predominantly breastfed or predominantly formula fed during the first 6 months of life. Breastfeeding was associated with a reduced risk of obesity after adjusting for a variety of potential confounding factors, including age, gender, stage of sexual maturation, energy intake, time spent watching television, physical activity levels, maternal BMI and other variables that reflect social, economic and lifestyle factors.
- The only study of the 8 that found no relationship between breastfeeding and obesity was by Wadsworth et al.[22] The researchers studied 3731 children 6 years of age in the United Kingdom after controlling for social class, birth weight, household crowding and fat intake at 4 years of age (but not for maternal overweight). This study differed from the others because it was a retrospective analysis of a cohort of children born in 1946, when the potential confounding factors of the relationship between breastfeeding and child overweight could have differed from the confounding factors in cohorts of children born more recently.

Results for Adolescents

Among the 7 studies of adolescents (or those studies that included children representing a wide range of ages, including adolescents), 3 showed a clear relationship between breastfeeding and reduced risk of overweight and 4 showed mixed or inconsistent results.

- A study by Kvaavik et al[23] of 635 adolescents 11 to 16 years of age in Norway reported a significant AOR of 0.15 for obesity in those breastfed for more than 3 months, compared to those adolescents who were never breastfed as infants.
- A paper by Kramer[24] reported on results from 2 separate studies. In both studies, the relative risk for overweight was much lower among adolescents who had been breastfed as infants, even after controlling for several confounding variables.
- Tulldahl and colleagues[25] studied older teenagers in Sweden. Among teens who had been exclusively breastfed for more than 2 months, 12.6% were overweight, compared to 17.9% of those who had been exclusively breastfed for ≤ 2 months. However, the investigators did not adjust for potentially confounding factors.
- Four studies on adolescents had mixed or inconsistent results:
  - A longitudinal study by Poulton and Williams[26] followed a cohort of more than 1000 children from 3 to 26 years of age. In the unadjusted results, breastfeeding for more than 6 months was associated with a lower risk of obesity at 9 to 18 years of age, but not at younger ages (3 to 7 years of age) or older ages (> 21 years of age). When controlling for maternal BMI and other confounding factors, the odds ratios at 9 to 18 years were of similar magnitude but no longer significant (most likely because the sample size was smaller because of missing data on maternal BMI for many of the subjects).
  - In a cross-sectional study of children 4 to 18 years of age from the UK by Li and colleagues,[27] there was no significant association between duration of breastfeeding and obesity, after adjusting for gender, parental BMI, maternal smoking, birth weight and social class.

- Victora et al[28] examined several indices of body composition among 2250 males 18 years of age in Brazil. Obesity was less likely in those adolescents who had been breastfed for 3 to 5 months, but the association was not significant for the other categories of breastfeeding duration (eg, > 5 months). However, there was a significant and linear decreasing trend of obesity with increased duration of *predominant* breastfeeding.
- Nelson and colleagues[29] studied the association between breastfeeding and overweight using data for 11,998 subjects from the U.S. National Longitudinal Study of Adolescent Health; the study included a subsample of 850 sibling pairs. In the full cohort, the odds of being overweight declined with increasing duration of breastfeeding, especially among girls. However, there was no evidence that breastfeeding had an effect on the risk of being overweight in the analysis of sibling pairs. The authors concluded that the significant association observed in the full cohort may have been because of residual confounding. One limitation of comparing siblings who were fed differently as infants is that the reason for not breastfeeding 1 member of a sibling pair may influence the outcome (eg, weight status). For example, 1 of the siblings may have had a health problem at birth that prevented breastfeeding and also led to slower weight gain, in which case any effect on overweight may be concealed. Thus, confounding can be an issue for both the full sample and the subgroup analyses.

Results From Meta-Analyses

There are also 2 meta-analyses on the association between breastfeeding and obesity.[30,31] One study,[30] which focused on childhood obesity, included 9 of the studies described above[13-17,20,21,26,27] and calculated an overall AOR for "ever breastfed" of 0.78, which was statistically significant. The second analysis,[31] which included all age ranges from infants to adults, reviewed 61 studies, 28 of which had odds ratio estimates. The unadjusted odds ratios (OR) for "ever breastfed" were significant for all age groups (OR = 0.50 for infants, OR = 0.90 for young children, OR = 0.66 for older children and OR = 0.80 for adults). After adjusting for socioeconomic status, parental BMI and maternal smoking, the AOR for the studies that included these covariates was still significant but was considerably weaker (AOR = 0.93; 95% confidence interval 0.88–0.99) than the unadjusted OR. However, the relationship between breastfeeding and reduced risk of obesity was stronger for "exclusive" breastfeeding (OR = 0.76) and for breastfeeding duration of ≥ 2 months (OR = 0.89). The authors did not calculate adjusted odds ratios for these more restrictive definitions of breastfeeding.

In general, the findings from these meta-analyses are limited by the variability across studies with regard to the definition of breastfeeding used (eg, categories of breastfeeding duration, and the degree of "exclusivity" of breastfeeding) and the number of covariates included in the analysis.

Influence of Duration and Exclusivity of Breastfeeding

Harder and colleagues[32] published a meta-analysis that examined whether there was a "dose-response" relationship between duration of breastfeeding and reduced risk of childhood obesity. They included 17 studies, and found that the OR for overweight declined as the duration of breastfeeding increased: Compared to breastfeeding for < 1 month, the OR for overweight for ≥ 7 months of breastfeeding was 0.67. However, these authors did not adjust for any potentially confounding variables in their analyses.

The influence of the exclusivity of breastfeeding on overweight was evaluated in the study by Bogen et al.[12] These authors examined the AOR for child overweight with increasing duration of breastfeeding (among white children whose mothers did not smoke during pregnancy), with and without supplementation with infant formula. Within each category of breastfeeding duration, the AOR was lower when there was no formula supplementation, after controlling for several covariates. For example, with > 26 weeks of breastfeeding, the AOR was 0.70 with formula supplementation and 0.55 without supplementation. Thus, a "dose-response" relationship has been observed with regard to both duration and exclusivity of breastfeeding.

Summary of Results Across All Studies

When comparing across studies with differing age ranges, or within the studies that were longitudinal, the association of overweight with breastfeeding appears strongest among school-aged children and adolescents, during the ages when there is rapid maturation and substantial fat deposition. This suggests that breastfeeding may have a "programming effect" that does not manifest itself fully until the preadolescent and adolescent growth spurts occur.

Potential Explanations for the Association Between Breastfeeding and Lower Risk of Child Overweight

There are 3 main categories of potential explanations for the association between breastfeeding and reduced risk of later obesity:

- Learned self-regulation of energy intake
- Metabolic programming
- Residual confounding by parental attributes and/or the family environment

Learned Self-Regulation of Energy Intake

One of the advantages of breastfeeding is that it allows the infant to control the amount of milk consumed, based on internal satiety cues. The mother does not know how much milk the infant has taken in, and cannot continue to feed the child if the child loses interest. By contrast, a bottle-fed infant may be encouraged to finish the bottle — even if already full — particularly if the caregiver has a predetermined idea of how much formula should be consumed, doesn't want to waste the formula, or believes that the child will be satisfied or sleep longer if more is consumed. One hypothesis is that this "overriding" of the infant's satiety cues during bottle feeding may lead to later difficulty with the ability to self-regulate energy intake.

In an experimental study, it was demonstrated that breastfed infants were able to self-regulate the amount of breast milk they consumed, provided that their mothers nursed on demand.[33] Other evidence for infant control of breast milk intake is the negative correlation between breast milk energy density (determined primarily by fat content) and milk intake of exclusively breastfed infants.[34,35] Infants whose mothers produce higher-fat milk generally consume less milk, presumably reflecting self-regulation to match their energy needs.

What is unknown is whether formula-fed infants are less able to self-regulate their intake than breastfed infants, and if so, whether these differences persist later in life. It is well documented that formula-fed infants consume more milk and gain weight more rapidly than breastfed infants, even in the first few months of life.[36] Interestingly, the difference in milk intake between breastfed and formula-fed infants becomes greater with age: At 1 month of age there is a relatively small difference in the mean volume consumed (< 100 mL/d), but by 5 months of age the difference is approximately 250 mL/d.[37] Furthermore, when solid foods are introduced, breastfed infants usually decrease the amount of breast milk consumed, whereas formula-fed infants continue to consume the same amount of formula, even as other foods are added to the diet.[38] These findings suggest that the self-regulatory ability of formula-fed infants worsens over time.

The long-term consequences of this phenomenon are unknown, but in studies of baboons, overfeeding in infancy leads to an increase in fat depot mass during puberty, especially among females.[39] In human studies,[40-42] rapid weight gain during infancy has been correlated with childhood obesity. In a study of 19,397 U.S. children born between 1959 and 1965,[41] the rate of weight gain during the first 4 months of life was strongly associated with the risk of obesity at 7 years of age, even after adjustment for weight status at 1 year of age. Almost 20% of childhood obesity was attributable to being in the top quintile for weight gain from birth to 4 months of age. The investigators did not have adequate data on infant feeding, so they could not examine the direct link between obesity and breastfeeding.

Stettler et al[43] attempted to identify the age interval during infancy that is the most sensitive period with regard to the relationship between early weight gain and adult overweight. They analyzed data for a sample of 653 formula-fed infants who were measured frequently during infancy and again at 20 to 32 years of age. As adults, 32% were overweight. Weight gain during the first week of life was the strongest predictor of adult overweight: The AOR for each 100-gram increase was 1.28 (range of 1.08 to 1.52), adjusted for gender, birth weight, type of formula, age at follow-up, maternal and paternal weight status, and income. In this sample, mean weight gain during the first week of life was 205 grams (ranging from 0 grams to 400 grams), whereas breastfed infants typically lose some weight in the first few days, with little or no net weight gain by 7 days. Thus, this very early difference in weight gain may have a long-term impact on later risk of obesity, perhaps through some sort of metabolic programming.

Metabolic Programming

There are several hormonal mechanisms by which infant feeding mode may affect child obesity:

- Plasma insulin levels can be influenced by mode of feeding. Formula-fed infants have been shown to have higher plasma insulin levels and a prolonged insulin response at 6 days of age, compared to breastfed infants,[44] and recent data indicate that the difference in plasma insulin is still apparent at 5 months of age.[37] Higher insulin levels stimulate greater adipose tissue deposition, and have been associated with subsequent increased weight gain and obesity in Pima Indian children 5 to 9 years of age.[45]

  One way that infant feeding mode may influence insulin levels is through protein intake. Formula-fed infants consume 66% to 70% more protein than breastfed infants at 3 to 6 months,[46] and by 12 months their intakes may be 5 to 6 times what is needed, depending on the types of complementary foods consumed. Higher protein intake tends to stimulate higher insulin secretion. An association between high protein intake in early life and overweight in childhood has been reported by some investigators,[47,48] but not all.[49] This issue requires further research to determine if there are any adverse consequences of high protein intake during infancy.[50] It may be that there are negative effects only at very high protein intakes.

- It has been suggested that breastfeeding may affect leptin metabolism during infancy and later in life, either via direct exposure to leptin in human milk, or indirectly via the effects of the rate of weight gain on leptin levels. Leptin is a key regulator of appetite and body fatness. Leptin levels tend to be positively correlated with body fatness, and higher leptin levels are thought to inhibit appetite unless there is "leptin resistance." A study by Singhal and colleagues[51] showed that the early diet of preterm infants is associated with plasma leptin concentration at 13 to 16 years of age. The ratio of leptin concentration to fat mass was lowest among children who had the highest consumption of human breast milk in early life. The investigators propose that greater body fatness during infancy programs the leptin-dependent feedback loop to be less sensitive to leptin later in life, leading to greater leptin resistance. In rats, there is evidence that overfeeding before weaning leads to overweight and leptin resistance at later ages.[52]

Residual Confounding by Parental Attributes and/or the Family Environment

Although biologic mechanisms for the relationship between breastfeeding and childhood obesity are plausible, we cannot yet rule out the possibility that the results of the studies described in the previous section are due to residual confounding by attributes of the parents and/or the family environment that were not measured. Most of the investigators attempted to control for as many confounding variables as possible. However, there are 2 variables in particular that are likely to be linked with breastfeeding, but are difficult to assess:

- Child feeding practices and parental control over feeding
- Physical activity

Child Feeding Practices and Parental Control Over Feeding

Fisher and colleagues[53] found that mothers who breastfed for at least 12 months reported using lower levels of "control" over feeding when their children were 18 months of age than did mothers who did not breastfeed as long. Similarly, Taveras et al[54] reported that a longer duration of breastfeeding was associated with less restrictive feeding behavior when the child was 12 months of age. Researchers have hypothesized that highly controlling feeding practices interfere with the child's ability to self-regulate energy intake, and there is some evidence to support this link.[55]

Physical Activity

Because parents who choose to breastfeed may have a healthier lifestyle in general, it is also possible that levels of physical activity are higher in these families: This may be the causal link between breastfeeding and child obesity. Five of the studies described in the previous section were able to control for the child's physical activity.[19,20,21,23,28] In these studies, the association between breastfeeding and lower rates of obesity remained significant when taking into account physical activity levels. Nonetheless, because it is difficult to assess a child's entire history of physical activity, residual confounding is still a concern.

As mentioned previously, a study by Nelson and colleagues[29] concluded that residual confounding was a likely explanation for the relationship between breastfeeding and obesity, based on their analysis of sibling pairs. Further research of this nature would be useful to sort out the extent to which unmeasured familial factors account for the lower rates of overweight among children who were breastfed.

Other Infant Feeding Behaviors That May Influence the Risk of Child Obesity

There are several infant feeding practices, apart from not breastfeeding, that may increase the risk of child overweight. They include the following:

- Bottle feeding that is not responsive to the infant's satiety cues
- Offering large volumes of formula
- Introducing solid foods at an early age
- Providing large amounts of juices or sweetened beverages

To date, the evidence regarding the influence of these practices is scanty. In a study comparing intake and growth of 52 exclusively breastfed and 84 formula-fed infants,[37] the associations between 2 specific bottle-feeding behaviors and infant growth were examined in the formula-fed cohort. The behaviors examined were the tendency for "bottle-emptying," defined as the percentage of feeds at which ≤ 10 mL of formula remained unconsumed, and the usual amount of formula prepared per feed (ie, "bottle size").

For the first behavior, mother-infant pairs were categorized in terms of whether they emptied the bottle frequently (≥ 50% of feeds) or infrequently (< 50% of feeds). Infants in the group that emptied the bottle more frequently had greater body fatness at 5 months of age (measured by sum of skinfold thickness, 69 vs 55 mm, $P<.01$).

For the second behavior, mothers were categorized in terms of whether they usually prepared ≤ 6 oz (180 mL) per feed or > 6 oz per feed when their infant was 3 months of age. The cut-off of 6 oz per feed for bottle size was chosen because it was observed that the breastfed infants in the study rarely consumed more than that amount at a single feed. The formula-fed infants who were usually offered bottles that contained > 6 oz of formula had significantly greater formula intake at 3 months of age than those infants who were regularly offered bottles that contained ≤ 6 oz of formula (1008 vs 785 mL/d, $P = .001$), even though there was no significant difference in intake in early infancy (at 1 month of age). There was also a significant difference in weight gain between 3 months of age and 5 months of age (21.0 vs 17.4 grams/day in the "larger bottle" vs "smaller bottle" groups, respectively, $P = .03$).

These results suggest that bottle feeding practices may encourage excess intake. However, in an observational study it is difficult to distinguish whether it is the caregiver's wishes or the infant's characteristics that are driving larger bottle size and bottle emptying. Thus, a randomized controlled intervention trial that is able to modify bottle-feeding behaviors by caregivers is needed to adequately test the hypothesis that these behaviors explain the differences in intake and growth between breastfed and formula-fed infants.

Early introduction of solid foods has been identified as a risk factor, independent of breastfeeding, for child obesity in some studies,[13,56,57] but not in others.[19,24] Breastfed infants may be able to compensate for the additional energy provided in solid foods by decreasing breast milk intake, thereby reducing any long-term impact of the age of introduction of such foods.

Consumption of fruit juices and sweetened drinks among preschool-aged children has also been associated with child obesity in the United States,[58,59] although the evidence is mixed.[60,61] The American Academy of Pediatrics, concerned about the effects of excessive juice consumption by infants, particularly when infants are bottle-fed juices, has issued statements discouraging the feeding of juice in a bottle to infants and advising limits on the consumption of juice among infants and preschool-aged children.[62]

Clinical and Public Health Implications and Intervention Strategies

Substantial evidence supports the link between breastfeeding and reduced risk for child obesity:

- Of the 21 studies reviewed in this chapter, 17 showed a lower risk of overweight or obesity among children who were breastfed, after controlling for potential confounding factors.[6,9,11-13,15-21,23-25,28,29]

- All of the studies that took into account the exclusivity of breastfeeding showed a significant association between breastfeeding and a lower rate of child overweight.[11-14,16,17,19,21,24,25,28]
- Of the 16 studies that controlled for maternal BMI, 13 showed a significant relationship.[6,9,12,13,15,18-21,23,24,25,28]

The significant adjusted odds ratios were generally in the range of 0.55 to 0.80, depending on the duration and exclusivity of breastfeeding. This indicates that the odds of being overweight or obese were about 20% to 45% lower in children who had been breastfed. A dose-response relationship was observed in a meta-analysis of studies with information on the duration of breastfeeding.

If the relationship between breastfeeding and child overweight is causal, the effect of breastfeeding is probably moderate when compared to other factors such as parental overweight, later dietary practices and physical activity. Nonetheless, its role in preventing child overweight could still be of significance given the epidemic of child obesity currently facing the United States. There has been progress in the United States in improving the rate of initiation of breastfeeding (currently close to 70%), but the average duration and exclusivity of breastfeeding are still far below national goals.[63] Thus, promotion of breastfeeding is a high priority, particularly exclusive breastfeeding during the first 6 months of life and continued breastfeeding, without formula supplementation, thereafter.

Successfully promoting breastfeeding requires multiple channels of action, including education, improving health services, legislation and services for employed mothers, mothers' support groups, and regulation and monitoring of the infant food industry. The target groups for educational campaigns include the general public (mass media campaigns, school curricula), pregnant women and their families (prenatal and postnatal education), and healthcare professionals (medical and nursing school curricula, continuing education activities, lactation management training courses and scientific meetings).

The Baby-Friendly Hospital Initiative, originated by UNICEF, is directed at improving healthcare services related to breastfeeding. Hospitals that provide maternity services are encouraged to adopt the "Ten Steps to Successful Breastfeeding," which involve training all hospital staff in the policies and skills needed to help mothers successfully initiate and maintain breastfeeding.[64] Several studies have demonstrated that adopting these 10 steps has a strong impact on rates of exclusive breastfeeding.[65,66] Unfortunately, to date, less than 2% of hospitals with maternity services in the United States have been certified as Baby-Friendly.[67] Much more progress can be made by encouraging all hospitals that provide maternity care to adopt model policies that promote breastfeeding.

Employment need not be a barrier to breastfeeding if adequate legislation and services for working mothers are in place. Legislation should include paid maternity leave for the first several months postpartum to allow mothers to successfully establish exclusive breastfeeding. Employers should establish worksite policies that accommodate breastfeeding through on-site day care, nursing breaks, flextime and the provision of lactation rooms where mothers can privately express and store their breast milk. Employers that provide such services can reap the benefits of net cost savings due to lower absenteeism and turnover among breastfeeding mothers, whose infants are typically healthier than infants not breastfed.[64]

Mothers' support groups, such as La Leche League, play a unique role by providing one-on-one peer support for breastfeeding mothers. Activities such as group meetings, maternity ward visits, house calls and phone advice are geared towards helping breastfeeding mothers initiate and maintain breastfeeding.

At the global level, regulation and monitoring of the infant food industry has been an important strategy to discourage inappropriate marketing of breast milk substitutes. The International Code of Marketing of Breastmilk Substitutes, adopted by the World Health Organization in 1981, includes 10 provisions regarding advertising and promotion of infant formulas. Although dozens of countries have made some or all of the code legally binding, the United States is not among them. Infant formula companies in the United States use marketing strategies that are in violation of the code, including advertising directly to the public and promoting their products via free supplies to hospitals, gift packs to mothers and other tactics.

Strategies that combine several of the above approaches, such as public education and improvement in healthcare services, are likely to be most effective at increasing breastfeeding rates. Several lessons have been learned from the many interventions that have been attempted[68-70]:

- One-on-one counseling has the most consistent positive effect. It is not sufficient to simply hand out a brochure or provide a video, as the barriers to breastfeeding vary greatly among mothers, and direct assistance to overcome certain breastfeeding difficulties often is needed.
- Peer counseling can be an effective intervention because mothers feel most empowered to breastfeed when there is a role model with whom they can identify, preferably from a similar cultural background.
- Involvement of the entire community, including men, is important. Negative social attitudes regarding breastfeeding in public, or the appropriate duration of breastfeeding, for example, can be a barrier for some mothers.
- Development of an early postpartum component to the breastfeeding intervention is essential, given the high percentage of mothers who have difficulties establishing breastfeeding in the first 1 to 2 weeks.
- Home visits by trained breastfeeding counselors during the early postpartum period are more effective than lactation clinics, presumably because the latter require that mothers have the time and transportation to get to the clinic.

Because other feeding behaviors can influence the risk of child obesity, as described in the previous sections of this chapter, a comprehensive strategy for promoting optimal infant feeding practices — which includes breastfeeding — should be developed. One potential approach is to train breastfeeding peer counselors to educate caregivers about infant feeding and assist them with developing and using responsive feeding practices, especially if they are bottle feeding their infants. Peer counselors should encourage caregivers to:

- Mimic the way breastfed infants feed (more frequent, smaller feeds than are typical with bottle feeding)
- Let the child determine how much to consume by being sensitive to early satiety cues
- Avoid encouraging the child to empty the bottle
- Avoid early introduction of solid foods
- Limit the amount of juices offered and avoid sweetened beverages such as soda

To be successful with this approach, it is essential to promote discussion of potential barriers to implementing the desired behaviors, including the influence of family and friends, concerns about infant crying and sleeping, and attitudes towards infant growth and fatness.

A parallel effort is needed to educate healthcare professionals to endorse and support these infant feeding messages. Healthcare providers must be trained not to overemphasize weight gain as the main indicator of adequate growth and development, and to include other indicators such as motor development. Assuring caregivers that an infant is thriving, rather than congratulating them on how much weight the child has gained, may help to change attitudes that "bigger is better" during infancy. Adoption of the new World Health Organization growth charts (released in April 2006), which are based on growth of breastfed children, will ensure that appropriate judgments about the adequacy of growth are made. Healthcare providers also need to be aware that despite a lower average weight-for-length among breastfed infants at 12 to 18 months of age, compared to formula-fed infants, some breastfed infants will still become overweight. Parents often are worried about this, and some clinicians go so far as to recommend reducing the number of breastfeeds. There is no evidence that this is effective, and it may in fact be counterproductive. Thus, current advice is that no intervention is needed, other than to assure that other feeding practices are appropriate and that the caregivers are responsive to the child's hunger and satiety cues.

The evidence to date suggests that breastfeeding reduces the risk of child obesity. If this relationship is indeed causal, it appears to be due to a latent effect of infant feeding mode, not solely to lower fatness during the first 2 years of life. The evidence regarding the effect of other infant feeding practices is limited and requires further research. Randomized intervention trials, for example, to evaluate the impact of training peer counselors to promote both breastfeeding and other optimal infant feeding practices, are an essential next step towards developing effective national strategies to reduce child obesity.

References

1. Baskin ML, Ard J, Franklin F, Allison DB. Prevalence of obesity in the United States. *Obesity Review.* 2005;6:5-7.
2. Wang Y. Cross-national comparison of childhood obesity: the epidemic and the relationship between obesity and socioeconomic status. *International Journal of Epidemiology.* 2001;30:1129-1136.

3. Dewey KG, Heinig MJ, Nommsen LA, Peerson JM, Lönnerdal B. Breast-fed infants are leaner than formula-fed infants at 1 year of age: the DARLING study. *American Journal of Clinical Nutrition.* 1993;57:140-145.
4. Dewey KG, Peerson JM, Brown KH, et al. Growth of breast-fed infants deviates from current reference data: a pooled analysis of US, Canadian and European data sets. *Pediatrics.* 1995;96:495-503.
5. Kalies H, Heinrich J, Borte M, et al. The effect of breastfeeding on weight gain in infants: results of a birth cohort study. *European Journal of Medical Research.* 2005;10:36-42.
6. Burke V, Beilin LJ, Simmer K, et al. Breastfeeding and overweight: longitudinal analysis in an Australian birth cohort. *Journal of Pediatrics.* 2005;147:56-61.
7. Baker JL, Michaelson KF, Rasmussen KM, Sorensen TIA. Maternal pre-pregnant body mass index, duration of breastfeeding and timing of complementary food introduction are associated with infant weight gain. *American Journal of Clinical Nutrition.* 2004;80:1579-1588.
8. Kramer MS, Guo T, Platt RW, et al. Feeding effects on growth during infancy. *Journal of Pediatrics.* 2004;145:600-605.
9. Grummer-Strawn LM, Mei Z. Does breastfeeding protect against pediatric overweight? Analysis of longitudinal data from the Centers for Disease Control and Prevention Pediatric Nutrition Surveillance System. *Pediatrics.* 2004;113:e81-e86.
10. Rasmussen KM, Hilson JA, Kjolhede. Obesity may impair lactogenesis II. *Journal of Nutrition.* 2001;131:3009S-3011S.
11. Armstrong J, Reilly JJ, Team CHI. Breastfeeding and lowering the risk of childhood obesity. *Lancet.* 2002;359:2003-2004.
12. Bogen DL, Hanusa BH, Whitaker RC. The effect of breast-feeding with and without formula use on the risk of obesity at 4 years of age. *Obesity Research.* 2004;12:1527-1535.
13. Hediger ML, Overpeck MD, Kuczmarski RJ, Ruan WJ. Association between infant breastfeeding and overweight in young children. *Journal of the American Medical Association.* 2001;285:2453-2460.
14. O'Callaghan MJ, Williams GM, Andersen MJ, Bor W, Najman JM. Prediction of obesity in children at 5 years: a cohort study. *Journal of Paediatrics and Child Health.* 1997;33:311-316.
15. Bergmann KE, Bergmann RL, Von Kries R, et al. Early determinants of childhood overweight and adiposity in a birth cohort study: role of breast-feeding. *International Journal of Obesity-Related Metabolic Disorders.* 2003;27:162-172.
16. von Kries R, Koltezko B, Sauerwald T, et al. Breast feeding and obesity: cross sectional study. *British Medical Journal.* 1999;319:147-150.
17. Liese AD, Hirsch T, von Muitius E, Keil U, Leupold W, Weiland SK. Inverse association of overweight and breast feeding in 9 to 10 year old children in Germany. *International Journal of Obesity.* 2001;25:1644-1650.
18. Li C, Kaur H, Choi WS, Huang TTK, Lee RE, Ahluwalia JS. Additive interactions of maternal prepregnancy BMI and breast-feeding on childhood overweight. *Obesity Research.* 2005;13:362-371.
19. Reilly JJ, Armstrong J, Dorosty AR, et al. Avon Longitudinal Study of Parents and Children Study Team: Early Risk Factors for Obesity in Childhood: Cohort Study. Available at: http://www.bmj.bmjjournals.com. Accessed August 9, 2006.
20. Toschke AM, Vignerova J, Lhotska L, Osancova K, Koletzko B, von Kries R. Overweight and obesity in 6- to 14-year old Czech children in 1991: protective effect of breastfeeding. *Journal of Pediatrics.* 2002;141:764-769.
21. Gillman MW, Rifas-Shiman SL, Camargo CA Jr, et al. Risk of overweight among adolescents who were breastfed as infants. *Journal of the American Medical Association.* 2001;285:2461-2467.
22. Wadsworth M, Marshall S, Hardy R, Paul A. Breast feeding and obesity: relation may be accounted for by social factors. *British Medical Journal.* 1999;319:1576.
23. Kvaavik E, Tell GS, Klepp KI. Surveys of Norwegian youth indicated that breast feeding reduced subsequent risk of obesity. *Journal of Clinical Epidemiology.* 2005;58:849-855.
24. Kramer MS. Do breast-feeding and delayed introduction of solid foods protect against subsequent obesity? *Journal of Pediatrics.* 1981;98:883-887.

25. Tulldahl J, Pettersson K, Andersson SW, Hulthen L. Mode of infant feeding and achieved growth in adolescence: early feeding patterns in relation to growth and body composition in adolescence. *Obesity Research.* 1999;7:431-437.
26. Poulton R, Williams S. Breastfeeding and risk of overweight. *Journal of the American Medical Association.* 2001;286:1449.
27. Li L, Parsons TJ, Power C. Breast feeding and obesity in childhood: cross sectional study. *British Medical Journal.* 2003;327:904-905.
28. Victora CG, Barros FC, Lima RC, Horta BL, Wells J. Anthropometry and body composition of 18-year-old men according to duration of breast feeding: birth cohort study from Brazil. *British Medical Journal.* 2003;327:901-905.
29. Nelson MC, Gordon-Larsen P, Adair LS. Are adolescents who were breast-fed less likely to be overweight? *Epidemiology.* 2005;16:247-253.
30. Arenz S, Ruckerl R, Koletzko B, von Kries R. Breast-feeding and childhood obesity: a systematic review. *International Journal of Obesity-Related Metabolic Disorders.* 2004;28:1247-1256.
31. Owen CG, Martin RM, Whincup PH, Davey Smith G, Cook DG. Effect of infant feeding on the risk of obesity across the life course: a quantitative review of published evidence. *Pediatrics.* 2005;115:1367-1377.
32. Harder T, Bergmann R, Kallischnigg G, Plagemann A. Duration of breastfeeding and risk of overweight: a meta-analysis. *American Journal of Epidemiology.* 2005;162:1-7.
33. Dewey KG, Lönnerdal B. Infant self-regulation of breast milk intake. *Acta Paediatrica Scandinavia.* 1986;75:893-898.
34. Nommsen LA, Lovelady CA, Heinig MJ, Lönnerdal B, Dewey KG. Determinants of energy, protein, lipid and lactose concentrations in human milk during the first 12 months of lactation: the DARLING study. *American Journal of Clinical Nutrition.* 1991;53:457-465.
35. Pérez-Escamilla R, Cohen RJ, Brown KH, Rivera LL, Canahuati J, Dewey KG. Maternal anthropometric status and lactation performance in a low-income Honduran population: evidence for the role of infants. *American Journal of Clinical Nutrition.* 1995;61:528-534.
36. Dewey KG. Growth characteristics of breast-fed compared to formula-fed infants. *Biology of the Neonate.* 1998;74:94-105.
37. Dewey KG, Nommsen-Rivers L, Lönnerdal B. Plasma insulin and insulin-releasing amino acid (IRAA) concentrations are higher in formula-fed than in breastfed infants at 5 months of age. Paper presented at: Experimental Biology 2004; April 20-24, 2004; Washington, DC.
38. Heinig MJ, Nommsen LA, Peerson JM, Lönnerdal B, Dewey KG. Intake and growth of breast-fed and formula-fed infants in relation to the timing of introduction of complementary foods: the DARLING study. *Acta Paediatrica.* 1993;82:999-1006.
39. Lewis DS, Bertrand HA, McMahan A, McGill HC, Carey KD, Masoro EJ. Pre-weaning food intake influences the adiposity of young adult baboons. *Journal of Clinical Investigation.* 1986;78:899-905.
40. Ong KKL, Ahmed ML, Emmett PM, Preece MA, Dunger DB. Association between postnatal catch-up growth and obesity in childhood: prospective cohort study. *British Medical Journal.* 2000;320:967-971.
41. Stettler N, Zemel BS, Kumanyika S, Stallings VA. Infant weight gain and childhood overweight status in a multicenter cohort study. *Pediatrics.* 2002;109:194-199.
42. Cameron N, Pettifor J, De Wet T, Norris S. The relationship of rapid weight gain in infancy to obesity and skeletal maturity in childhood. *Obesity Research.* 2003;11:457-460.
43. Stettler N, Stallings VA, Troxel AB, et al. Weight gain in the first week of life and overweight in adulthood: a cohort study of European American subjects fed infant formula. *Circulation.* 2005;111:1897-1903.
44. Lucas A, Boyes S, Bloom R, Aynsley-Green A. Metabolic and endocrine responses to a milk feed in six-day-old term infants: differences between breast and cow's milk formula feeding. *Acta Paediatrica Scandinavia.* 1981;70:195-200.

45. Odeleye OE, de Courten M, Pettitt DJ, Ravussin E. Fasting hyperinsulinemia is a predictor of increased body weight gain and obesity in Pima Indian children. *Diabetes.* 1997;46:1341-1345.

46. Heinig MJ, Nommsen LA, Peerson JM, Lönnerdal B, Dewey KG. Energy and protein intakes of breast-fed and formula-fed infants during the first year of life and their association with growth velocity: the DARLING study. *American Journal of Clinical Nutrition.* 1993;58:152-161.

47. Rolland-Cachera MF, Deheeger M, Akrout M, Bellisle F. Influence of macronutrients on adiposity development: a follow-up study of nutrition and growth from 10 months to 8 years of age. *International Journal of Obesity.* 1995;19:573-578.

48. Scaglioni S, Agostini C, Notaris RD, et al. Early macronutrient intake and overweight at 5 years of age. *International Journal of Obesity.* 2000;24:777-781.

49. Dorotsy AR, Emmett PM, Cowin S, Reilly JJ, Team AS. Factors associated with early adiposity rebound. *Pediatrics.* 2000;105:1115-1118.

50. Koletzko B, Broekaert I, Demmelmair H, et al. Protein intake in the first year of life: a risk factor for later obesity? The EU childhood obesity project. *Advances in Experimental Medical Biology.* 2005;569:69-79.

51. Singhal A, Farooqi IS, O'Rahilly S, Cole TJ, Fewtrell M, Lucas A. Early nutrition and leptin concentrations in later life. *American Journal of Clinical Nutrition.* 2002;75:993-999.

52. Plagemann A, Harder T, Rake A, et al. Observations on the orexigenic hypothalamic neuropeptide Y-system in neonatally overfed weanling rats. *Journal of Neuroendocrinology.* 1999;11:541-546.

53. Fisher JO, Birch LL, Smiciklas-Wright H, Picciano MF. Breast-feeding through the first year predicts maternal control in feeding and subsequent toddler energy intakes. *Journal of the American Dietetic Association.* 2000;100:641-646.

54. Taveras EM, Scanlon KS, Birch L, Rifas-Shiman SL, Rich-Edwards JW, Gillman MW. Association of breastfeeding with maternal control of infant feeding at age 1 year. *Pediatrics.* 2004;114:e577-e583.

55. Birch LL, Fisher JO, Davison KK. Learning to overeat: maternal use of restrictive feeding practices promotes girls' eating in the absence of hunger. *American Journal of Clinical Nutrition.* 2003; 78:215-220.

56. Baker JL, Michaelson KF, Rasmussen KM, Sorensen TIA. Maternal pre-pregnant body mass index, duration of breastfeeding, and timing of complementary food introduction are associated with infant weight gain. *American Journal of Clinical Nutrition.* 2004;80:1579-1588.

57. Wilson AC, Forsyth JS, Greene SA, et al. Relation of infant diet to childhood health: seven year follow up of cohort of children in Dundee infant feeding study. *British Medical Journal.* 1998;316: 21-25.

58. Dennison BA, Rockwell HL, Baker SL. Excess fruit juice consumption by preschool-aged children is associated with short stature and obesity. *Pediatrics.* 1997;99:15-22.

59. Welsh JA, Cogswell ME, Rogers S, Rockett H, Mei Z, Grummer-Strawn LM. Overweight among low-income preschool children associated with the consumption of sweet drinks: Missouri, 1999-2002. *Pediatrics.* 2005;115:e223-e229.

60. Newby PK, Peterson KE, Berkey CS, Leppert J, Willett WC, Colditz GA. Beverage consumption is not associated with changes in weight and body mass index among low-income preschool children in North Dakota. *Journal of the American Dietetic Association.* 2004;104:1086-1094.

61. Alexy U, Sichert-Hellert W, Kersting M, Manz F, Schoch G. Fruit juice consumption and the prevalence of obesity and short stature in German preschool children: results of the DONALD Study. *Journal of Pediatric Gastroenterology and Nutrition.* 1999;29:343-349.

62. American Academy of Pediatrics, Committee on Nutrition. The use of fruit juice in the diets of young children. *American Academy of Pediatrics News.* Feb 1991;7:2.

63. Li R, Zhao A, Mokdad A, Barker L, Grummer-Strawn L. Prevalence of breastfeeding in the United States: the 2001 National Immunization Survey. *Pediatrics.* 2003;111:1198-1201.

64. Shealy KR, Li R, Benton-Davis S, Grummer-Strawn LM. *The CDC Guide to Breastfeeding Interventions.* Atlanta, Ga: U.S. Department of Health and Human Services, Centers for Disease Control and Prevention, 2005.

65. Kramer MS, Chalmers B, Hodnett ED, et al. For the PROBIT Study Group. Promotion of breastfeeding intervention trial (PROBIT): a randomized trial in the Republic of Belarus. *Journal of the American Medical Association.* 2001;285:413-420.

66. Cattaneo A, Buzzetti R. Effect on rates of breastfeeding of training for the Baby-Friendly Hospital Initiative. *British Medical Journal.* 2001;323:1358-1362.

67. Radford A, Saadeh R, Labbok MH. Meeting on Baby-Friendly Hospital Initiative. *Standing Committee on Nutrition News.* 2004;28:54-56.

68. Couto de Oliveira MI, Camacho LAB, Tedstone AE. Extending breastfeeding duration through primary care: a systematic review of prenatal and postnatal interventions. *Journal of Human Lactation.* 2001;17:326-343.

69. Anderson AK, Damio G, Young S, Chapman DJ, Perez-Escamilla R. A randomized trial assessing the efficacy of peer counseling on exclusive breastfeeding in a predominantly Latina low-income community. *Archives of Pediatric Adolescent Medicine.* 2005;159:836-841.

70. Sikorski J, Renfrew MJ, Pindoria S, Wade A. Support for breastfeeding mothers: a systematic review. *Paediatric Perinatal Epidemiology.* 2003;17:407-417.

Section 2
Cultural and Parenting Influences

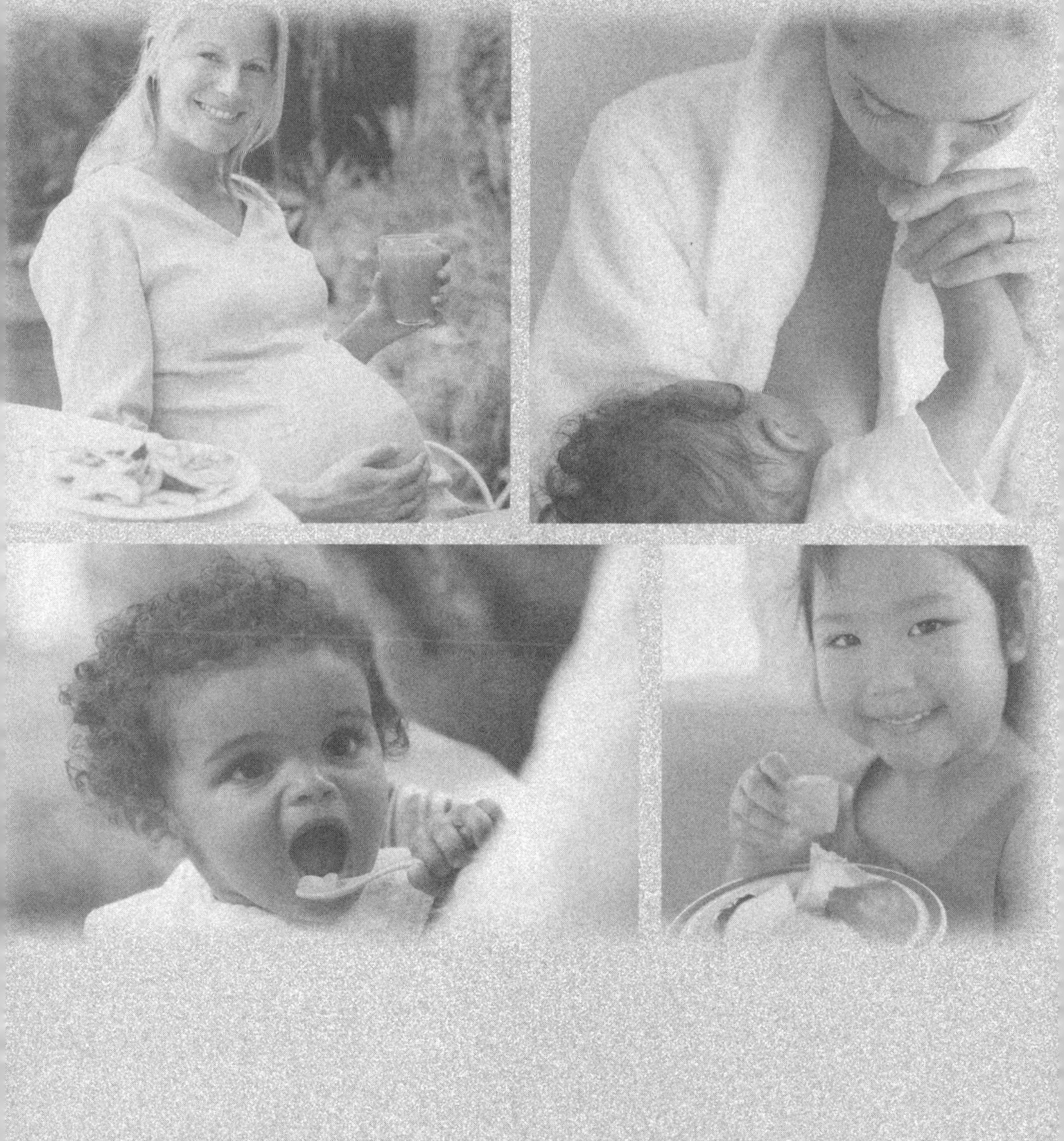

Abstracts From Section 2 Cultural and Parenting Influences

Linking Television Viewing and Childhood Obesity

Elizabeth A. Vandewater, PhD

Youth of all ages spend more time daily using electronic media than pursuing any other single leisure-time activity except for sleep. Recent surveys confirm the general perception that children are growing up in media- and technology-saturated environments. Partly because children spend so much time using electronic media, healthcare providers, public health experts, educators, policymakers and others have labeled it a culprit in the rising obesity rates among US children. If television can be implicated in the childhood obesity epidemic in this country, then public health experts and scholars need to understand just how it is implicated — as well as the ways in which it is not. The evidence clearly suggests that televised advertising for high-fat and sugared foods is one likely mechanism through which TV viewing affects childhood obesity.

Dietary Intakes of Infants and Toddlers: Problems Start Early

Barbara Devaney, PhD
Mary Kay Fox, MEd

The first 2 years of a child's life are a period of rapid physical, cognitive, emotional and social development. During this critical time, parents and caregivers make many important decisions about what, when and how to feed their children. Over the past several years, through analysis of data from the Feeding Infants and Toddlers Study (FITS), sponsored by Gerber Products Company in 2002, much has been learned about the nutrient adequacy of infant and toddler diets, foods consumed, timing and sequence of the introduction of table foods, transitions in infant and toddler diets, portion size and energy intake, among other topics. There is some good and some not-so-good news from these study findings. The good news is that most infants and toddlers are getting enough vitamins and minerals to meet their requirements for healthy growth and development. The not-so-good news is that infants and toddlers appear to be getting too many calories and, as they transition from infant foods to table foods, some problematic eating patterns emerge. This chapter summarizes key findings from the FITS analyses.

Feeding Children in an Environment of Plenty: Lessons From the Laboratory

Jennifer Orlet Fisher, PhD
Leann L. Birch, PhD

For most of human history, children ate in conditions of scarcity, with much of family life devoted to the procurement and preparation of food. Today, in non-Third World countries, children's eating habits evolve under conditions of dietary abundance. Food and drink are available in most venues of everyday life. The increasing presence of overweight and obesity among children in the United States and other developed countries suggests that limited food resources are no longer a pressing threat to child health. Traditional feeding concerns and strategies — that developed in response to food scarcity — may be ineffective or even counterproductive under conditions of plenty. Children's food preferences and their diets reflect the foods that are available and accessible to them in part because familiarity drives preference. This chapter reviews research indicating that young children are exposed to conditions of dietary excess through the ecology of the family eating environment.

Do Race and Ethnicity Influence Parents' Feeding Strategies, Perceptions of and Concerns About Child Weight, and Intervention Techniques?

Bettylou Sherry, PhD, RD
Kelley S. Scanlon, PhD, RD
Elizabeth Barden, PhD
Jan Kallio, MS, RD, LDN

As the prevalence of pediatric obesity continues to increase, healthcare professionals are challenged to address this important public health problem. A growing body of evidence suggests that parents' feeding strategies, specifically strategies that restrict what a child eats, may actually contribute to overeating and to a child becoming overweight. Little research exists, however, on the impact of race and ethnicity on feeding strategies and the association between race/ethnicity and children's food intake and weight. Understanding cultural influences on feeding practices, parental perceptions of, and concerns about, children's weight, and strategies for motivating change can enhance the design of interventions aimed at improving children's diets and reducing pediatric obesity. This chapter reviews the available research on these issues, which includes focus-group studies and quantitative analyses.

Linking Television Viewing and Childhood Obesity

Elizabeth A. Vandewater, PhD

Introduction

The prevalence of obesity among American youth has reached alarming levels. The percentage of overweight children and adolescents, as defined by a body mass index (BMI) exceeding the 95th percentile for age- and gender-based norms, has tripled over the past 3 decades.[1] Current estimates indicate that approximately 10% of children 2 to 5 years of age and 15% of children 6 to 19 years of age are overweight.[2]

Being overweight or obese has dire consequences for children's health. Overweight and obese children are at increased risk of suffering comorbidities, including type 2 diabetes, hypertension, dyslipidemia, hyperinsulinemia, fatty liver disease and orthopedic disorders.[3] Some 60% of overweight children have at least one cardiovascular risk factor (eg, hypertension, hyperlipidemia)[4] and the number of youth with some degree of glycemic abnormalities (precursors to type 2 diabetes mellitus) is on the rise — and closely parallels the trend in increasing weight status of youth globally.[5,6]

Moreover, overweight in childhood tends to persist into adulthood.[7] Overweight youth enter adulthood with a risk of obesity that is up to 17 times that of their normal-weight peers.[8] It has been estimated that obesity-related morbidity accounts for approximately 6% of national health expenditure in the United States.[9] Therefore, it is likely that the significant increase in the prevalence of overweight and obesity among children over the last three decades will dramatically affect public health expenses, programs and priorities well into the 21st century.

The Contemporary Children's Media Landscape

Youth of all ages spend more time daily using electronic media (for example, 3 to 5 hours a day watching television) than pursuing any other single leisure-time activity except for sleep.[10] Recent surveys confirm the general perception that children are growing up in media- and technology-saturated environments. Almost 100% of American households report that they own a television; roughly 75% reporting that they own more than one.[11] Increasingly, these televisions are located in children's bedrooms. Recent surveys indicate that 70% of children 8 to 18 years of age and 36% of very young children (6 months to 6 years of age) have televisions in their bedrooms.[11,12]

Computer and video game use among children also is growing: About 40% of youth 8 to 18 years of age report that they use computers or play video games on a daily basis.[11] However, survey data reveal that neither video game use nor computer use is nearly as ubiquitous or time-consuming as is television watching. Data collected in 2002 from a representative sample of American children ages 6 to 18 indicate that youth still spend far more time watching TV than they do playing electronic games and/or using computers, excluding games (HM Cummings, EA Vandewater, unpublished data, 2006). (See Figure 1.) These findings are similar to the findings from the Kaiser Family Foundation media surveys reported in 1999 and again in 2005.[11,13]

Television Viewing and Childhood Obesity: Is There a Link?

Partly because children spend so much time using electronic media, health-care providers, public health experts, educators, policymakers and others have labeled it a culprit in the rising obesity rates among U.S. children. The lay public and scholars alike blame television viewing specifically.[14-17] This perception now is shaping prominent public health policies. The American Academy of Pediatrics (AAP) has recommended that pediatricians advise parents to discourage television viewing for children under 2 years of age, and to limit the viewing time of older children to less than 2 hours a day.[18] In its continuing series of Healthy People mission statements, the United States Department of Health and Human Services listed the reduction of TV viewing as a national health objective for the first time in *Healthy People 2010.*

Figure 1. Children's media landscape in 2002.

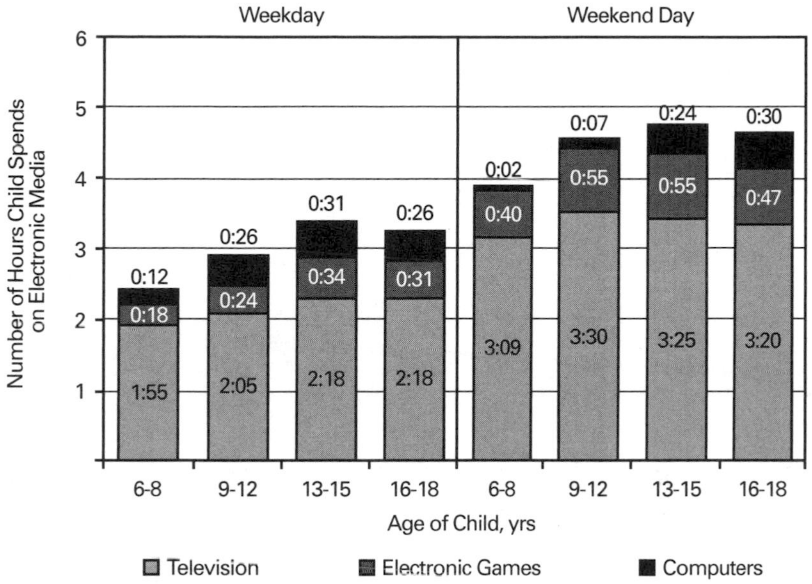

Charting Television Viewing and Childhood Obesity Over Time

The public, healthcare providers, public health experts and academicians alike generally believe that children's television viewing has increased over the years and commonly express the view that childhood obesity has increased along with it.[14] The theory that children's television viewing time has increased in proportion to and side by side with increases in childhood obesity is so commonly held that many scholars simply make the assertion, without offering supporting empirical evidence.

In reality, TV viewing among children in the United States has remained fairly steady over the past 3 decades (see Figure 2). Using estimates of viewing time from various sources, including estimates from my work and that of my colleagues,[19-23] I have charted the time children spent viewing television from the 1970s through 2002 against the prevalence of childhood obesity based

Figure 2. Prevalence of child overweight and television viewing over the past 30 years.

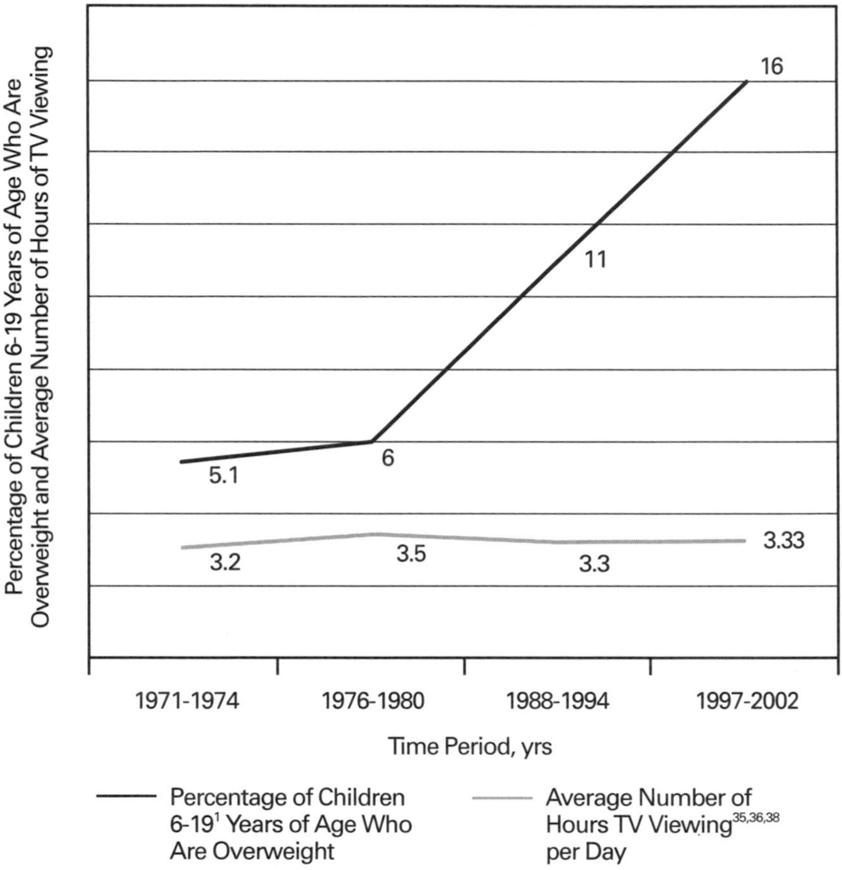

upon estimates from the National Health and Nutrition Examination Survey (NHANES) for the same time periods.[24-26] NHANES is a survey conducted annually by the Centers for Disease Control and Prevention to assess the health and nutritional status of adults and children in the United States. The data indicate that children in the United States watch 3 to 3.5 hours of television each day, and that this viewing level has remained steady since the mid-1970s. Carter examined the media use of Australian children in 1960 and 2003 and saw little change as well.[27] Childhood obesity rates, on the other hand, have climbed over this time period. In fact, after 1980, they began to rise sharply. Although 3.5 viewing hours daily is still a sizable amount of time spent in front of a television, it does not appear to be true that children's TV viewing has increased proportionately with the rise in childhood obesity.

Clearly children are watching a lot of television. But what exactly is the link between television viewing and obesity? Three major mechanisms are hypothesized to underlie the relationship between television viewing and obesity.[28] These mechanisms are:

- Decreased metabolic rates during television viewing
- Displacement of physical activity by the more sedentary behavior of watching television
- Increased caloric intake either through eating while watching television, or in response to televised food advertisements

Decreased Metabolic Rates

This hypothesis suggests that television viewing actually decreases resting metabolic rates in viewers to levels that are below the resting metabolic rates registered during other sedentary activities. If this were the case, then energy expenditure during television viewing would be lower than it is when sleeping or reading — and, therefore, television viewing should be discouraged. At the most fundamental level, this hypothesis posits that there is something about watching television itself that increases adiposity. This idea was first suggested by Eck and colleagues in 1992,[29] when they found evidence that the metabolic rates of children 8 to 12 years of age were lower during television viewing than during resting or sleeping. Although these findings received a lot of press at the time, they have generally proven unreplicable.[30,31] The current consensus in the field is that this is not a viable hypothesis.[28]

Decreased Activity Levels

Television and electronic media are commonly thought to contribute to weight gain in children because the time children spend engaging in these sedentary activities displaces energy-expending physical activity. This is essentially the "couch potato" hypothesis, and it is by far the most popular hypothesis connecting television use and obesity in children. It applies equally well to interactive media such as video games and computers. This hypothesis assumes that if a child were not watching television or playing an electronic game, he or she would be physically active — playing outdoors or riding a bicycle.

If the time a child spends in activities is zero-sum, then it makes intuitive sense that time spent watching television takes away from time available for more physically active activities. This is the known as "displacement effect."[32] However, it is worth noting that empirical examination of displacement or time "trade-offs" requires a full accounting of all the activities a child engages in over a 24-hour period. Otherwise, it is impossible to accurately assess the extent of the relationships among the activities in which children engage.[33] This realization is far from recent. In 1977, Robinson remarked: "A major weakness of the available literature has been its failure to employ an adequate sampling framework of daily life with which to assess television's full impact."[34] Yet, few studies use an appropriate time-sampling method. Given that concern about the displacement of healthier activities by television viewing has loomed large in both popular and academic consciousness for decades, the relative dearth of empirical research using this method is surprising.

Early evidence of television viewing displacing physical activity came from studies documenting decreases in participation levels in physical activities following the introduction of television into small, mainly rural communities.[35,36] Researchers found lower levels of participation in sports activities among both children and adults in rural communities that had access to either a single television channel or multiple television channels, compared to a community with no television.[36]

However, other epidemiologic studies have consistently found a small or nonexistent relationship between television viewing and physical activity among children and adolescents. Robinson and colleagues,[37] as well as DuRant and colleagues,[38] reported a weak negative correlation between television viewing and physical activity. Robinson and Killen[39] found no relationship between physical activity and television viewing. In a study conducted with my colleagues using time diaries to assess the relationship between television viewing and various activities (the only study that I am aware of that uses an appropriate time-sample method for examining displacement), we also found no relationship between television viewing and physical activity.[23]

Even Robinson's 1999 randomized controlled experiment that found reductions in children's adiposity with reductions in television viewing did not find commensurate changes in physical activity.[40] Therefore, although Robinson's findings provide solid evidence supporting the theory that reducing television time can reduce adiposity in children, the mechanism linking television viewing with childhood obesity remained open to interpretation. In a recent meta-analysis, Marshall and colleagues[41] examined findings from 52 independent samples and reported an average effect size (Pearson *r*) of -.12. Though this relationship is in the predicted direction, the size of the relationship is extremely small. The authors concluded that "…media-based inactivity may be unfairly implicated in recent epidemiologic trends of overweight and obesity among children and youth."[41]

Thus, while it may be generally assumed that if children are not watching television, they would be outside running up and down a soccer field, existing evidence does not support this assumption. In fact, it seems that television viewing mainly displaces other kinds of sedentary activities. In our research, we found that increases in television viewing were correlated with decreases in time spent in other indoor pastimes, including board games, pretend play, card games and other relatively sedentary activities.[23] Thus, the current body of empirical evidence suggests that television viewing does not contribute to childhood overweight and obesity by replacing strenuous physical activity.

If a decrease in physical activity levels is not the mechanism by which television affects weight in children – what's left? Consider Figure 2 again. The divergence in obesity rates and TV viewing over the last 30 years suggests that something else is happening during viewing that is related to obesity other than the inactivity inherent in watching television. Which brings us to the third major hypothesized mechanism — that television viewing is linked to increased caloric intake, either because of eating that occurs while viewing, or in response to food advertising on television, which more often than not pitches high-calorie, high-fat foods with poor nutritional content.[42]

Increased Caloric Intake

Few empirical efforts to date have been aimed at directly assessing the idea that children and adults eat "mindlessly" while watching television. Coon and colleagues examined the nutritional content of foods consumed by a sample of children in grades 4 through 6 (n = 91) from families who reported whether or not the television was on during the 3 main meals of the day.[43]

Overall, they found that the children whose families ate 2 or more meals in front of the television each day derived 6% more of their total daily energy intake from the meat group, 5% more from pizza, salty snacks and sodas combined, and nearly 5% less from fruits, vegetables and juices combined.[43] Interestingly, they also found that *added* fats were consumed less often by children in these same families, perhaps because these children were eating fattier foods to begin with — one rarely adds butter to pizza.

In a similar study of a sample of ethnically diverse children in grades 3 through 5 (n = 60), Matheson and colleagues[44] found that food was consumed more often while viewing TV than during any other activity. On average, 75% of children ate while viewing television on the weekdays, and 60% ate while watching on the weekends. Overall, the children were more likely to consume snacks than any other foods while watching television. Beyond these trends, the results were inconsistent. Depending on the day of the week and the grade level of the child, children were either more or less likely to consume soda or fruit while watching television. It is notable, however, that regardless of the day of the week or the grade level of the child, vegetables were less likely than any other food to be consumed during television viewing.[44]

Both of these studies are based on small, community-based samples, and therefore cannot be generalized to the population of children and adolescents in the United States. Utilizing the same data set referenced in Figure 1 (HM Cummings, EA Vandewater, unpublished data, 2006), my colleagues and I examined eating while viewing television using time-diary data in a broader population: a representative sample of 2569 children and adolescents 5 years of age to 18 years of age in the United States. Overall, we found that 35% of the children ate their meals in front of the television at least once on a weekday, and 37% of the children did so on a weekend day. These numbers are considerably lower than those reported by Matheson and colleagues,[44] perhaps because of sample differences, cohort differences or some other differences. Though intriguing, the findings from all of these studies do not definitively answer the question of whether television viewing promotes caloric consumption. The notion of "mindless" eating implies that either individuals eat more than they normally would during meals consumed in front of the television, or that television viewing provides additional opportunities to eat aside from meals. As of yet, these subtleties have not been put to any empirical test. Clearly, more research on this issue is needed using a variety of designs and methods (eg, experimental, epidemiological, longitudinal).

Televised Food Advertising

After the automotive industry, the United States food industry is the second largest advertiser in the American economy.[45] In 1997, the US Department of Agriculture spent $333 million on nutrition education, evaluation and demonstrations.[46,47] By contrast, the food industry spent $7 billion on food advertising in 1997.[46] Nearly one-third of this expenditure ($2.3 billion) was for advertising that promoted confectionary foods and snacks, breakfast cereals and soft drinks.

Children are an increasingly important market for advertisers. In the past decade in particular, US children and adolescents have been targeted with increasingly intensive and aggressive forms of food advertising [48,49] For the food industry, the stakes are huge. In 1998, McNeal estimated that children 14 years of age and younger directly purchased $14 billion in goods annually, and influenced another $190 billion in family purchases.[50] With the advent of cable television and direct broadcast satellite, and the resulting proliferation of television channels, there are now numerous channels with programming aimed specifically at children, including Nickelodeon, Disney Channel and Cartoon Network.[51] The concentration of particular demographics among the viewers of these "niche" channels makes it easier for advertisers to target specific markets, including children.

By 2002, food and beverage advertisers spent $10 billion to $12 billion collectively on messages aimed at children and youth.[52] Of that, approximately $1 billion is spent on media advertising to children — primarily through television.[51,52] Advertisers spend approximately $1 billion annually on messages aimed at youth, and television is the preferred mode of reaching them.[51,53,54]

In the United States, more than 75% of the advertising budgets of food manufacturers and 95% of the advertising budgets of fast food restaurants are allocated to TV advertising.[47] Food is one of the most frequently advertised products on television and accounts for almost half of all commercials during children's programming.[55,56]

The average American child watches more than 40,000 television commercials per year and commercial advertising has been found to account for as much as 16% of children's total viewing time.[57] A recent content analysis showed that 30% of advertising for a child audience was for food products.[58]

It has been estimated that children are exposed to an average of 1 food commercial for every 5 minutes of television viewing.[59] If children watch an average of 3 hours of TV per day and each commercial averages 30 seconds, they may view more than 2 hours of food commercials every week.

Food manufacturers advertise frequently to children, especially young children, because of their desire to develop and build brand awareness, preference and loyalty early on.[48] Hite and Hite demonstrated that food preferences in young children (especially very young children from 2 to 3 years of age) are driven largely by "branding."[58] They found that young children evaluated the product samples that had nationally advertised brand names and/or labels as tasting significantly better than did products with store names and/or labels.[58] Children who were 2 to 3 years of age chose brand names/labels 10 to 1 over store names/labels, while children 4 to 5 years of age chose brand names/labels 2 to 1 over store names/labels.[58]

These findings have not gone unnoticed by food marketers, who have been intensifying their efforts to develop brand relationships with young consumers.[60] Some 80% of all food items are branded,[46] and marketers know that very young children can affect parental purchases through what is called as the "nag factor" or "pester power."[48,50] Marketers also know that a child's first request for a product occurs at around 2 years of age, and that 75% of the time this request occurs in a grocery store or supermarket. Among the first-time, in-store requests by children, the most frequently requested item is breakfast cereal (47%), followed by snacks and beverages (30%), and toys (21%).[48,50]

Television food advertising directed at children falls mostly into the following 5 categories: 1) pre-sugared breakfast cereals, 2) soft drinks, 3) candy, 4) salty snack products, and 5) fast food and/or highly processed foods.[61] In 1994, Kotz and Story constructed a "Saturday Morning Food Pyramid" that illustrated the types and frequencies of food advertising to children.[61] They found that 50.3% of foods advertised during children's television programs could be categorized as fats, oils and sweets; 43.4% as bread, cereal, rice and pasta; 4.5% as dairy; and 1.8% as meat, poultry, fish, eggs, nuts and legumes. Thus, sweets made up the majority of the "Saturday Morning Pyramid," and vegetables and fruits were completely absent — the antithesis of the US Department of Agriculture's Food Guide Pyramid at the time.[61] A more recent analysis of food advertising during programming to children in 2003 revealed that convenience/fast foods and sweets (including candy and soft-drinks) comprised 83% of the advertised foods.[58]

Children's Comprehension of Advertising

A plethora of evidence suggests that young children have difficulty making sense of commercials and commercial content:

- Children under 4 years of age have difficulty differentiating between programs and commercials[62]
- Children under 7 years of age do not understand the persuasive intent of advertising — they are more likely to perceive ads as "information" provided by someone with their best interests at heart[63]
- Even children between the ages of 7 and 11 have difficulty questioning commercial claims[64]

Often, the language in TV commercials that provides important information about the product is presented in ways children cannot understand. For example, children under 7 years of age do not understand the meaning of the words "part of a balanced breakfast," which almost ubiquitously is used in sugared cereal advertisements.[65] As noted by Kunkel and colleagues, "Rather than informing young viewers about the importance of a nutritious breakfast, this common disclaimer actually leaves many children with the misimpression that cereal alone is sufficient for a meal."[51]

Features of Advertising to Children

Market researchers and advertisers have spent a great deal of time, effort and money trying to understand how to appeal most effectively to children.[64] Advertising to children commonly includes music, quick-cut editing (to speed up the pace of the ad), sound effects and animation — which are all used because they can capture a child's attention.[66] Television advertisers have also learned to repeat ads frequently during children's programming based on research findings that show that repetition is an effective teaching strategy, especially for young children.[64] In addition, marketers now know that products are most appealing when they presented in terms of "fun."[67]

The most common persuasive strategy employed in advertising targeted at children is to associate the product with fun and happiness.[68,69] Popular and well-liked cartoon characters are used often in advertising directed to children because they enhance children's ability to recall the product and their product preference.[70,71] Using a character in a television advertisement that is featured in adjacent programming is a practice known as "host-selling." For example, an ad for Cocoa Pebbles cereal featuring Fred Flintstone that aired during a commercial break from the Flintstones cartoon program would be considered host-selling.[57] Host-selling is a particularly powerful practice because it muddies the waters even further when children — especially young children — attempt to differentiate between programming and advertising.[72] Because of this, the Federal Communications Commission (FCC) has restricted the practice during children's programming.[73]

Effects of Food Advertising on Children

There is little doubt that the diets of American children and adolescents are nutritionally inadequate and often do not meet national dietary goals.[73-75] Moreover, US food consumption data show some shifts over the past few decades:

- Children and adolescents are eating more food away from home, drinking more soft drinks and snacking more frequently[77,78]
- American children now obtain more than 50% of their daily calories from fat (32%) or added sugar (20%)[79]
- Do these shifts have anything to do with the heavy marketing of such foods to children?

Researchers have sought to answer this question by examining the impact of advertising on children's food preferences, requests to parents for food products and parental purchases of food products.[50,56,80-83] Coon and Tucker reviewed the literature and came to the following conclusions[84]:

- Evidence from experimental studies consistently shows that exposure to advertisements for food products increases children's choice of and preference for such products
- Exposure to televised food advertising increases children's requests to parents for the purchase of the advertised food items

- The frequency of children's requests to purchase specific brands or categories of food products is positively correlated with the frequency of the advertising for these products

From the perspective of marketers at least, it appears that food advertising to youth works and it works well.

Because our primary concern is to understand the mechanism by which television may lead to childhood obesity, the *critical* question is whether televised food advertising actually increases children's consumption of advertised foods. The answer to this question is somewhat harder to come by. Only a few studies have been conducted on the effects of food advertising on children's food intake, in part because of the inherent difficulties in controlling children's exposure to advertising and foods outside of experimental settings.[84]

Gorn and Goldberg conducted a now-classic study that examined the effect of exposure to televised snack food commercials on children's actual food consumption.[85] Children 5 to 8 years of age attending a summer camp viewed daily for 2 weeks a 30-minute cartoon with roughly 5 minutes of embedded food advertising. The types of advertising were varied to create 4 experimental conditions, exposing the children to: 1) candy and Kool-Aid® ads; 2) fruit and fruit juice ads; 3) public service ads for healthy foods; 4) no ads (the control group). Each day after the television exposure, the children were offered a snack and could choose from a selection of fruits, juices, candy or Kool-Aid. Children in the group that viewed advertisements for candy and Kool-Aid chose candy as their snack more frequently than did children in the group that viewed advertisements for fruits and fruit juices. In addition, children who viewed candy and Kool-Aid ads chose fruit and juice as a snack less frequently than did children in any other group.[85]

Hitchings and Moynihan found that consumption of advertised foods by children 9 to 11 years of age was positively correlated (between .50 and .60) with their ability to recall food advertisements as assessed by food diaries maintained over a 3-day period.[86] Another study examined recognition of food advertising and consumption of specific foods by children in response to advertising and found that overweight and obese children recognized more ads and ate more of the advertised foods following experimental exposures to food advertising than did normal-weight children.[87] However, all children in this study, regardless of their weight, ate more of the advertised food following exposure to televised advertising than did children in a control group that did not view the food advertising.[87]

Though there are limitations to the existing research, on the whole, the evidence implicates televised food advertising as a mechanism that links television viewing with increases in childhood obesity. A recent report by the World Health Organization and the Food and Agriculture Organization of the United Nations rated the strength of existing evidence linking dietary and lifestyle factors to obesity as "convincing," "probable," "possible" or "insufficient." The report concluded that there is enough sufficient indirect evidence that advertising of fast food restaurants and energy-dense, nutrient-poor food and beverages to children causes obesity to place it in the "probable" category.[88]

Promoting Healthy Food Choices: Finding Hope in Public Service Announcements

There is little doubt that children are susceptible to advertising, and their food preferences, food choices and food intake are shaped by their exposure to it. Since children learn the things they are taught, then we should also be able to influence children's food preferences and consumption in more desirable ways through advertising of healthy foods and healthy eating behaviors.

Various studies have demonstrated that children shown ads for healthy products or pro-nutritional public service announcements (PSAs) chose more fruits and juices as snacks than did those children who viewed ads for sugared products,[85] ate fewer sugared foods in a post-viewing test[89] and scored higher on nutritional knowledge tests.[90] Recently, Sesame Workshop™ has been exploring whether the appeal of well-known Sesame Street® characters could increase children's preferences for fruits and vegetables if fruits and vegetable were somehow tied to these characters. They found that placing a favorite Muppet character sticker on foods increased children's preferences for those foods, and that placing a character sticker on a healthier food (eg, broccoli) could increase children's preference for that food over a less healthy choice (eg, a chocolate bar) that did not have the character sticker placed on it.[91] These findings suggest that the simple placement of stickers depicting popular and well-known characters on healthier foods could play an important role in increasing the appeal of healthy foods for children.[91] Because it is easier to reinforce children's preferences for sweet and/or high-fat foods,[92,93] these findings are good news indeed.

Implications for Parents and Practitioners

The messages children glean from advertising and any behaviors that stem from these messages are affected by characteristics of the contexts in which they are exposed — whether at home, in school or with their friends. Children do not grow and learn in a vacuum, and their responses to advertising, in general, and food advertising, in particular, can be shaped significantly by parents and peers. Children learn from their parents how to respond to media messages, and parents can shape the nature of their children's responses to advertising, a process known as "parental mediation."[94,95] The take-home message children get from the media can be changed considerably through parent-child discussions of the message.[96]

Because of the level of media saturation in our society, it is inevitable that children will see food advertising, or that they will hear about "cool" new foods from friends who have been exposed to advertisements. However, access and availability to food items are necessary for children's consumption. This is why interest groups and parents have fought so hard to remove soft drinks and fast foods from schools, on the one hand, and why fast-food restaurants, on the other hand, often are located within walking distance of schools. Parents provide (or give their approval for) the majority of the food that children 10 years of age and under consume. Therefore, although televised food advertising will increase children's requests for food items, parents don't have to purchase these foods or bring them into the home.

One of the most insidious aspects of marketing is that advertising in general has become "normalized." Many parents set limits regarding the content of the programs that their children may watch,[97] but few would rush over to turn off the television set during a commercial. Pediatricians and other healthcare providers should inform parents that food commercials are far from benign. Parents should be encouraged to resist their children's requests for nutritionally poor food and to use videos or DVDs for their children's allotted television viewing because they often contain less advertising — product placement notwithstanding. Finally, PSAs aimed at influencing children's nutritional knowledge can borrow from the advertising literature and use techniques known to improve the efficacy of the message.

Implications for Research

If television can be implicated in the childhood obesity epidemic in this country, then public health experts and scholars need to understand just how it is implicated — as well as the ways in which it is not. Overall, the relationship between television viewing and childhood obesity, though perhaps not as strong as had been assumed, is evident in enough studies to warrant concern. The difficulty lies in uncovering the *reason* for this relationship. To date, there is little evidence that television viewing displaces other more physical activities among children. However, there are serious limitations to existing research in this area. For example, existing studies did not examine possible moderating influences such as ethnicity or neighborhood characteristics, so that it is unclear whether the relationship between television and activity level (and childhood obesity) might be different for different groups of children (which would tend to "wash out" the effect at the population level). In addition, there is a dearth of longitudinal studies that track the relationship between television viewing and activity levels as children grow.

In contrast, the evidence does clearly suggest that televised advertising for high-fat and sugared foods is one likely mechanism through which TV viewing affects childhood obesity. Yet there are limitations to existing research in this area as well. The majority of studies that examine the impact of food advertising on children's food preferences and behaviors were conducted in the mid 1970s and 1980s. To date, no meta-analysis that looks at the size of the effect of food advertising on children's food preferences, food choices, food intake or purchase requests exists, and prospective longitudinal studies are likewise absent. There is a particular need for research on the relationship between advertising and caloric intake, as well as how the content and impact of food advertising varies by ethnic group.

Conclusions

In this paper, I reviewed the evidence for the possible major mechanisms linking television viewing and childhood obesity. Given the depth and strength of popular and scholarly convictions that television viewing plays a role in the increased prevalence of obesity in children, the supporting evidence is surprisingly equivocal. There are many possible explanations for this:

- Moderating factors may be at work, which would mean that these relationships are strong for some children and nonexistent for others
- Inexact measurement of media use, caloric intake, activity level or all three may be hampering the ability to detect relationships
- Perhaps the relationships unfold over longer periods of time (years rather than months), which would require longer-term longitudinal studies
- Perhaps TV viewing is simply a marker of other things, such as the social isolation of obese adolescents, or poor parenting in general — including providing nutritionally poor food for children

As childhood obesity is a very real threat to public health, it is crucial to identify the central factors that contribute to its development so that we may then appropriately target prevention and intervention efforts. It seems safe to say that media — including television and computer games — play an ever increasing role in our daily lives. Therefore, gaining a thorough understanding of the nature of media's impact on health and well-being should be a vital component of the public health agenda in the United States and other developed nations.

Acknowledgment

Funding for this research was provided by Grant R01-HD40851-01 from the National Institute of Child Health and Human Development, and population center grant 5-R24-HD42849 from the National Institute of Child Health and Human Development.

References

1. Troiano R, Flegal K. Overweight children and adolescents: description, epidemiology, and demographics. *Pediatrics.* 1998;101:497-504.
2. Ogden CL, Carroll MD, Curtin LR, McDowell MA, Tabak CJ, Flegal KM. Prevalence of overweight and obesity in the United States, 1999-2004. *Journal of the American Medical Association.* 2006;295:1549-1555.
3. Must A, Spadano J, Coakley EH, Field AE, Colditz G, Dietz WH. The disease burden associated with overweight and obesity. *Journal of the American Medical Association.* 1999;282:1523-1529.
4. Freedman DS, Dietz WH, Srinivasan SR, Berenson GS. The relation of overweight to cardiovascular risk factors among children and adolescents: the Bogalusa Heart Study. *Pediatrics.* 1999;103:1175-1182.
5. Bloomgarden ZT. Type 2 diabetes in the young: the evolving epidemic. *Diabetes Care.* 2004;27:998-1010.

6. Lobstein T, Baur L, Uauy R. International Obesity Task Force for the obesity in children and young people: a crisis in public health. Report to the World Health Organization. *Obesity Reviews.* 2004;5 (suppl.1):4-104.
7. Must A. Morbidity and mortality associated with elevated body weight in children and adolescents. *American Journal of Clinical Nutrition.* 1996:445S-447S.
8. Hauner H. Transfer into adulthood. In: Kiess W, Marcus C, Wabitsch M, eds. *Obesity in Childhood and Adolescence.* Vol 9. Basel, Switzerland: Karger; 2004:219-228.
9. Wolf A, Colditz GA. Current estimates of the economic cost of obesity in the United States. *Obesity Research.* 1998;6:97-106.
10. Huston AC, Wright JC. Mass media and children's development. In: Siegel I, Remminger A, vol eds; Damon W, series ed. *Handbook of Child Psychology.* 5th ed. New York, NY: John Wiley & Sons; 1997:999-1058.
11. Kaiser Family Foundation. *Generation M: Media in the Lives of 8-18 Year Olds.* Menlo Park, Calif: Kaiser Family Foundation; 2005.
12. Kaiser Family Foundation. *The Media Family: Electronic Media in the Lives of Infants, Toddlers, Preschoolers and Their Parents.* Menlo Park, Calif: Kaiser Family Foundation; 2006.
13. Kaiser Family Foundation. *Kids and Media @ The New Millennium.* Menlo Park, Calif: Kaiser Family Foundation; 1999.
14. Chen JL, Kennedy E. Television viewing and children's health. *Journal of the Society of Pediatric Nursing.* 2001;6:35.
15. Dietz WH. The obesity epidemic in young children: reduce television viewing and promote playing. *British Medical Journal.* 2001;322:313-314.
16. Dietz WH, Gortmaker SL. Do we fatten our children at the television set? Obesity and television viewing in children and adolescents. *Pediatrics.* 1985;75:807-812.
17. Gortmaker SL, Must A, Perrin JM, Sobol AM, Dietz WH. Social and economic consequences of overweight in adolescence and young adulthood. *New England Journal of Medicine.* 1993;329: 1008-1012.
18. American Academy of Pediatrics. Committee on Public Education. Children, adolescents and television. *Pediatrics.* 2001;107:423-426.
19. Lyle J, Hoffman HR. Children's use of television and other media. In: Rubinstein EA, Comstock GA, Murray JP, eds. *Television and Social Behavior: Vol. 4. Television in Day-to-Day Life: Patterns of use.* Washington, DC: Government Printing Office; 1972.
20. Comstock G, Chaffee S, Katzman N, Maxwell M, Roberts D. *Television and Human Behavior.* New York, NY: Rand Corporation; 1978.
21. *National Audience Demographics Report.* New York, NY: AC Nielson; 1976.
22. Timmer SG, Eccles J, O'Brien K. How children use time. In: Juster FT, Stafford FP, eds. *Time, Goods, and Well Being.* Ann Arbor, Mich: Institute for Social Research, University of Michigan; 1985: 353-369.
23. Vandewater EA, Bickham DS, Lee JH. Time well spent? Relating media use to children's free-time activities. *Pediatrics.* 2006;117:e181-e185.
24. Flegal KM, Carrol MD, Ogden CL, Johnson CL. Prevalence and trends in obesity among US adults, 1999-2000. *Journal of the American Medical Association.* 2002;288:1723-1727.
25. Ogden CL, Troiano RP, Briefel RR, Kuczmarski RJ, Flegal KM, Johnson CL. Prevalence of overweight among preschool children in the United States, 1971 through 1994. *Pediatrics.* 1997;99:1-7.
26. National Center for Health Statistics. *Chartbook on Trends in the Health of Americans.* Hyattsville, Md: National Center for Health Statistics; 2004.
27. Carter O. Changes in obesity, sedentary behaviours and Perth children's television viewing from 1960 to 2003. *Australian and New Zealand Journal of Public Health.* 2005;29:235.
28. Robinson TN. Television viewing and childhood obesity. *Childhood and Adolescent Obesity.* 2001;48: 1017-1025.

29. Eck LH, Klesges RC, Hanson CL, Slawson D. Children at familial risk for obesity: an examination of dietary intake, physical activity and weight status. *International Journal of Obesity.* 1992;16:71-78.
30. Buchowski MS, Sun M. Energy expenditure, televison viewing and obesity. *International Journal of Obesity and Related Metabolic Disorders.* 1996;20:236-244.
31. Dietz WH, Bandini LG, Morelli JA, Peers KF, Ching P. Effect of sedentary activities on resting metabolic rate. *Pediatrics.* 1994;59:556-559.
32. Mutz DC, Roberts DF, van Vuuren DP. Reconsidering the displacement hypothesis: television's influence on children's time use. *Communication Research.* 1993;20:51-75.
33. Juster FT, Stafford FP, eds. *Time, Goods, and Well-being.* Ann Arbor, Mich: Institute for Social Research, University of Michigan; 1985.
34. Robinson JP. *How American's Use Time: A Social-psychological Analysis of Everyday Behavior.* New York, NY: Praeger; 1977.
35. Brown JR, Cramond JK, Wilde RJ. Displacement effects of television and the child's functional orientation to media. In: Blumler J, Katz E, eds. *The Uses of Mass Communications: Current Perspectives on Gratifications Research.* Beverly Hills, Calif: Sage; 1974:93-112.
36. Williams TM, ed. *The Impact of Television: A Natural Experiment in Three Communities.* Orlando, Fla: Academic Press; 1986.
37. Robinson TN, Hammer LD, Killen JD, et al. Does televison viewing increase obesity and reduce physical activity?: Cross-sectional and longitudinal analyses among adolescent girls. *Pediatrics.* 1993;91:273-280.
38. DuRant RH, Baranowski T, Johnson M, Thompson WO. The relationship among televison watching, physical activity, and body composition of young children. *Pediatrics.* 1994;94:449-455.
39. Robinson TN, Killen JD. Ethnic and gender differences in the relationships between television viewing and obesity, physical activity, and dietary fat intake. *Journal of Health Education.* 1995;26:S91-S98.
40. Robinson TN. Reducing children's television viewing to prevent obesity: A randomized controlled trial. *Journal of the American Medical Association.* 1999;282:1561-1567.
41. Marshall SJ, Biddle SJH, Gorley T, Cameron N, Murdey I. Relationships between media use, body fatness and physical activity in children and youth: a meta-analysis. *International Journal of Obesity.* 2004;28:1238-1246.
42. Story M, Faulkner P. The prime time diet: a content analysis of eating behavior and food messages in television program content and commercials. *American Journal of Public Health.* 1990;80:738-740.
43. Coon KA, Goldberg J, Rogers BL, Tucker K. Relationships between use of television during meals and children's food consumption patterns. *Pediatrics.* 2005;107. Available at http://www.pediatrics.org/cgi/content/full/107/1/e7. Accessed July 2, 2006.
44. Matheson DM, Dillen JD, Wang Y, Varady A, Robinson TN. Children's food consumption during television viewing. *American Society for Clinical Nutrition.* 2004;79:1088-1094.
45. McCall KL. What's the big dif?: Differences between marketing and advertising. http://www.marketingprofs.com/preview.asp?file=/2/mccall5.asp. Accessed October 3, 2005.
46. Harris JM, Kaufman P, Martinez S, Price C. The US Food Marketing System, 2002. Washington, DC: Economic Research Service, US Department of Agriculture; 2002, Agricultural Economic Report No. 811.
47. Gallo AE. Food Advertising in the United States. In: Frazao E, ed. *America's Eating Habits: Changes and Consequences.* Washington, DC: US Department of Agriculture; 1999:173-180.
48. Story M, French S. Food advertising and marketing directed at children and adolescents in the US. *International Journal of Behavioral Nutrition and Physical Activity.* 2004;1:3-20. Available at http://www.ijbnpa.org/content/l/l/3.
49. Institute of Medicine. *Food Marketing to Children and Youth: Threat or Opportunity?* Washington, DC: National Academies Press; 2006.
50. McNeal J. Tapping the three kids' markets. *American Demographics.* 1998;20(4):37-41.

51. Kunkel D, Wilcox BL, Cantor J, Palmer E, Linn S, Dowrick P. *Report of the APA Task Force on Advertising and Children.* Washington, DC: American Psychological Association; 2004.
52. Institute of Medicine, Committee on the Prevention of Obesity in Children and Youth. *Preventing Childhood Obesity: Health in the Balance.* Washington, DC: National Academies Press; 2005.
53. Rice F. Superstars of spending: marketers clamor for kids. *Advertising Age*; 2001:S1.
54. Lauro PW. Coaxing the smile that sells: baby wranglers in demand in marketing for children. *The New York Times.* 1999:C1.
55. Dietz WH. Factors associated with childhood obesity. *Nutrition.* 1991;7:290.
56. Taras HL, Gage M. Advertised foods on children's television. *Archives of Pediatric and Adolescent Medicine.* 1995;149:649-652.
57. Kunkel D. Children and television advertising. In: Singer DG, Singer JL, eds. *The Handbook of Children and Media.* Thousand Oaks: Sage; 2001:375-394.
58. Hite CF, Hite RE. Reliance on brand by young children. *Journal of the Market Research Society.* 1994;37:185-193.
59. Gamble N, Cotunga N. A quarter century of TV food advertising targeted at children. *American Journal of Health Behavior.* 1999;23:261-267.
60. Zollo P. *Wise Up to Teens: Insight into Marketing and Advertising to Teenagers.* 2nd ed. Ithaca, NY: New Strategist Publications, Inc; 1999.
61. Kotz K, Story M. Food advertisements during children's Saturday morning television programming: are they consistent with dietary recommendations? *Journal of the American Dietetic Association.* 1994;94:1296-1301.
62. Ward S, Reale G, Levinson D. Children's perceptions, explanations, and judgements of television advertising: a further exploration. In: Rubinstein EA, Comstock GA, Murray JP, eds. *Television and Social Behavior.* Vol. 4. Television in Day-to-Day Life: Patterns of Use. Washington, DC: U.S. Government Printing Office; 1972:468-490.
63. Ward S, Wackman D, Wartella E. *How Children Learn to Buy: The Development of Consumer Information Processing Skills.* Beverly Hills, Calif: Sage Publications; 1977.
64. Kuribayashi A, Roberts MC, Johnson RJ. Actual nutritional information of products advertised to children and adults on Saturday. *Children's Health Care.* 2001;30:309-322.
65. Palmer E, McDowell C. Children's understanding of nutritional information presented in breakfast cereal commercials. *Journal of Broadcasting.* 1981;25:295-301.
66. Huston AC, Wright JA. Television forms and children. In: Comstock G, ed. *Public Communication and Behavior.* Vol 2. New York, NY: Academic Press; 1989:103-159.
67. Cantor J. Modifying children's eating habits through television ads: effects of humorous appeals in a field setting. *Journal of Broadcasting.* 1981;25:37-47.
68. Barcus FE. The nature of television advertising to children. In: Palmer E, Dorn D, eds. *Children and the Faces of Television.* New York, NY: 1981:273-285.
69. Kunkel D, Gantz W. Children's television advertising in the multi-channel environment. *Journal of Communication.* 1992;42:134-152.
70. Atkin C, Block M. Effectiveness of celebrity endorsers. *Journal of Advertising Research.* 1983;23: 57-61.
71. Lieber L. *Commercial and Character Slogan Recall by Children Aged 9 to 11 Years: Budweiser Frogs Versus Bugs Bunny.* Berkeley, Calif: Center on Alcohol Advertising; 1998.
72. Kunkel D. Children and host-selling television commercials. *Communication Research.* 1988;15: 71-92.
73. Kunkel D, Gantz W. Assessing compliance with industry self-regulation of television advertising to children. *Journal of Applied Communication Research.* 1993;21:148-162.
74. Cavadini C, Siega-Riz AM, Popkin BM. US adolescent food intake trends from 1965 to 1996. *Western Journal of Medicine.* 2000;173:378-383.

75. Nicklas TA, Elkasabany A, Srinivasan SR, Berenson G. Trends in nutrient intake of 10-year-old children over two decades (1973-1994): the Bogalusa Heart Study. *American Journal of Epidemiology.* 2001;153:969-977.

76. Neumark-Sztainer D, Story M, Hannan PJ, Croll J. Overweight status and eating patterns among adolescents: where do youths stand in comparison with the Healthy People 2010 objectives? *American Journal of Public Health.* 2002;92:844-851.

77. Jahns L, Siega-Riz AM, Popkin BM. The increasing prevalence of snacking among US children from 1977 to 1996. *Journal of Pediatrics.* 2001;138:493-498.

78. Gleason P, Suitor C. *Children's Diets in the Mid 1990's: Dietary Intake and its Relationship with School Meal Preparation.* Alexandria, Va: US Dept of Agriculture, Food and Nutrition Service; 2001. CN-01-CD1.

79. Gleason P, Suitor C. *Food for Thought: Children's Diets in the 1990s.* Princeton, NJ: Mathematica Policy Research, Inc; 2001.

80. Taras H, Zive M, Nader P, Berry CC, Hoy T, Boyd C. Television advertising and classes of food products consumed in a paediatric population. *International Journal of Advertising.* 2000;19:487-493.

81. Taras HL, Sallis JF, Patterson TL, Nader PR, Nelson JA. Television's influence on children's diet and physical inactivity. *Journal of Development and Behavioral Pediatrics.* 1989;10:176-180.

82. Borzekowski DLG, Robinson TN. The 30 second effect: an experiment revealing the impact of television commercials on food preferences of preschoolers. *Journal of the American Dietetic Association.* 2001;101:42-46.

83. Isler L, Popper HT, Ward S. Children's purchase requests and parental responses: results from a diary study. *Journal of Advertising Research.* 1987;27:28-39.

84. Coon KA, Tucker K. Television and children's consumption patterns. A review of the literature. *Minerva Pediatrica.* 2002;54:423-436.

85. Gorn GJ, Goldberg ME. Behavioral evidence for the effects of televised food messages to children. *Journal of Consumer Research.* 1982;9:200-205.

86. Hitchings E, Moynihan PJ. The relationship between television food advertisments recalled and actual foods consumed by children. *Journal of Human Nutritian and Dietetics.* 1998;11:511-517.

87. Halford JCG, Gillespie J, Brown V, Pontin EE, Dowling H. Effect of television advertisements for foods on food consumption in children. *Appetite.* 2004;42 221-225.

88. World Health Organization. *Joint WHO/FAO Expert Consultation on Diet, Nutrition and the Prevention of Chronic Disease.* Geneva, Switzerland: World Health Organization; 2003.

89. Galst J, White M. The unhealthy persuader: the reinforcing value of television and children's purchase influence attempts at the supermarket. *Child Development.* 1976;47:1089-1096.

90. Sylvester GP, Achterberg C, Williams J. Children's television and nutrition: friends or foes? *Nutrition Today.* 1995;30:6-14.

91. Cohen DI, Kotler JA, Royer SR. Preschoolers' perceptions of healthy food. *Society for Research in Child Development.* Atlanta, Ga; 2005.

92. Birch LL. Children's preferences for high-fat foods. *Nutrition Review.* 1992;50:249-255.

93. Birch LL. Development of food preferences. *Annual Review of Nutrition.* 1999;19:41-62.

94. Corder-Bolz CR. Mediation: the role of significant others. *Journal of Communication.* 1980;30: 106-118.

95. Fujioka Y, Austin EW. The implications of vantage point in parental mediation of television and child's attitudes toward drinking alcohol. *Journal of Broadcasting and Electronic Media.* 2003;45: 221-240.

96. Hogan MJ. Parents and other adults: models and monitors of healthy media habits. In: Singer DG, Singer JL, eds. *Handbook of Children and the Media.* Thousand Oaks, Calif: Sage; 2001:663-680.

97. Vandewater EA, Park SE, Huang X, Wartella EA. "No—you can't watch that": parental rules and young children's media use. *American Behavioral Scientist.* 2005;48:608-623.

Dietary Intakes of Infants and Toddlers: Problems Start Early

Barbara Devaney, PhD
Mary Kay Fox, MEd

Introduction

The first 2 years of a child's life are a period of rapid physical, cognitive, emotional and social development. During this critical time, parents and caregivers make many important decisions about what, when and how to feed their children. These decisions affect the nutritional quality of children's diets in infancy and childhood, and also may have a long-term impact on their food preferences and eating habits.[1-7]

The Feeding Infants and Toddlers Study (FITS), sponsored by Gerber Products Company in 2002, provides a comprehensive picture of the food and nutrient intakes of American infants and toddlers and of the feeding practices used by children's caregivers.[8,9] FITS fills this important gap in our knowledge base because existing national nutrition surveys have small samples of infants and toddlers under 2 years of age and, consequently, cannot support detailed assessments of this age group.[9] In addition, FITS was the first national survey to include contributions from dietary supplements in estimates of usual nutrient intakes and the first to use *Dietary Reference Intakes* to assess the adequacy and quality of usual intakes.[10-15]

FITS included a sample of infants and toddlers 4 to 24 months of age. Parents and caregivers of participating children completed up to 3 separate interviews, all conducted by telephone from March to July 2002. These interviews included:

- A brief recruitment and household interview
- A 24-hour dietary recall, with a supplemental set of questions on infant and toddler growth, development milestones, and feeding patterns and diet transitions

- A second 24-hour dietary recall interview for a random subsample of respondents

Over the past several years, through analysis of the FITS data, much has been learned about the nutrient adequacy of infant and toddler diets, the foods and beverages being fed, the timing and sequence of the introduction of table foods, transitions in infant and toddler diets, average portion sizes, energy intakes and other topics. Detailed results from FITS were published in 2 supplements to the *Journal of the American Dietetic Association* (January 2004 and January 2006).[8,9]

There is some good and some not-so-good news from these study findings. The good news is that most infants and toddlers are getting enough vitamins and minerals to meet their requirements for healthy growth and development. The not-so-good news is that infants and toddlers appear to be getting too many calories and, as they transition from infant foods to table foods, some problematic eating patterns emerge.[16-19] This chapter summarizes key findings from the FITS analyses about the energy intake and food consumption patterns of infants and toddlers.

Are Infants and Toddlers Consuming Too Many Calories?

FITS compared infants' and toddlers' reported usual energy (calorie) intakes with accepted standards, which are expressed as estimated energy requirements (EERs). The EER for an individual infant or toddler was defined as the calories required to maintain energy balance, given his or her age and weight, plus an allowance for the growth of the infant or toddler.[14] To assess whether energy intakes were too high or too low, means and distributions of reported usual energy intakes were compared with means and distributions of EERs.

In the FITS analysis, usual energy intakes of both infants and toddlers exceeded EERs, and the discrepancy between intakes and requirements increased with age (see Table 1).[16]

- For infants 4 to 6 months of age, the mean usual energy intake was about 10% greater than the mean EER

Table 1. Usual Energy Intakes and Estimated Energy Requirements of Infants and Toddlers

	Percentiles (kcal)			
	25th	**Median**	**Mean**	**75th**
Infants 4 to 6 months of age				
Usual intake	589	670	690	762
EER	562	622	629	683
Infants 7 to 11 months of age				
Usual intake	772	884	912	1021
EER	649	729	739	810
Toddlers 1 to 2 years of age				
Usual intake	1046	1220	1249	1419
EER	828	931	950	1050

Data are from 2002 Feeding Infants and Toddlers Study.[16]

EER = estimated energy requirement

Adapted from *Journal of the American Dietetic Association*, V104, S14-S21, Devaney B, Ziegler P, Pac S, Karwc V, Barr SI, Nutrient intakes of infants and toddlers, ©2004, with permission from The American Dietetic Association

- For infants 7 to 11 months, the mean usual energy intake was 23% greater than the mean EER
- For toddlers 12 to 24 months of age, the mean usual energy intake was 31% greater than the mean EER

The finding from FITS that energy intakes exceed EERs is consistent with findings from other studies.[20,21] A recent report from the Institute of Medicine Committee to Review the WIC [Women, Infants, and Children] Food Packages also found that energy intakes exceeded requirements for infants and children participating in WIC.[20] In addition, a recent report assessing the nutrient intakes of vulnerable subgroups reported that energy intakes of young children exceeded their requirements.[21] FITS estimates of energy intakes are consistent with published estimates from the third National Health and Nutrition Examination Survey and the Continuing Survey of

Food Intake by Individuals (CSFII), 1994-1996.[22,23] For example, for toddlers 12 to 24 months of age, the FITS estimate of usual calorie intake was 1244 kilocalories (kcal) per day and the CSFII estimate was 1256 kcal per day.[23]

There are 3 possible reasons why reported energy intakes in infants and toddlers may exceed EERs:

- Infants and toddlers may actually be consuming too many calories
- Parents and caregivers may have overreported food intakes
- EERs may have been underestimated

Although the increasing prevalence of overweight and obesity among children is consistent with an excess consumption of calories, the discrepancy in the FITS data between reported energy intakes and EERs is implausibly high, especially for toddlers (the mean energy intake among toddlers exceeded the EER by about 300 kcal per day).[16] Excessive calorie intakes of this magnitude would lead to weight gain of at least 1 pound every 2 weeks, or 25 pounds per year.

The fact that this rate of weight gain has not been observed suggests that the discrepancy between energy intakes and EERs may be at least partially due to parents or caregivers overreporting children's food intakes. Although the FITS data-collection methods included visual aids and extensive prompts to help parents estimate the quantities of foods consumed by their child, parents may have overreported intakes. Overreporting of food consumption for infants and toddlers may reflect an unconscious desire on the part of parents to characterize their children as good eaters. This raises an interesting question: Does the social desirability of having a good eater lead to actual overfeeding of infants and toddlers?

The third possible reason for the discrepancy between energy intakes and requirements — underestimation of calorie requirements — could occur if parents do not report their infant's weight correctly. Assuming that weight is assessed at well-baby visits to a doctor or clinic, it is probable that most children would have gained weight between the time they were last measured and the date of the FITS interview. Using higher weights in the EER calculations would have resulted in higher EERs and, therefore, a smaller difference between the EER and reported energy intakes. For example, a difference in weight of 1 kg (2.2 pounds) would increase the EER by 89 kcal.[14]

Relationship Between Portion Size and Energy Intake

Several researchers have hypothesized that increases in the size of typical food portions could be contributing to the obesity epidemic.[24,25] Initially, it may seem tautological that larger portion sizes lead to higher energy intakes. However, portion size is only one factor that contributes to total energy intake. Other factors that influence energy intake include the number of eating occasions in a day, the number of foods consumed and the energy density of the foods consumed. The extent to which portion size influences energy intake may vary depending on whether and how these other determinants of energy intake change as portion sizes change.

Infants have an innate ability to self-regulate energy intake, with intake being driven primarily by responses to hunger and satiety cues.[26-30] Research has demonstrated, however, that this innate ability deteriorates over time as eating becomes more influenced by external cues, such as palatability, schedule/routine and social context.[26,31,32] It is not known how early in life the deterioration of energy self-regulation begins.

To examine this issue, we used FITS data to look at the effects of portion size, number of eating occasions, number of foods consumed and energy density on energy intakes and then examined how portion size varied with these other predictors of energy intakes. (The ideal analysis would assess the relationship between portion size and weight-for-height. We were unable to look at this relationship, however, because of questionable reliability of the heights reported by caregivers.) To compare portion sizes across children, we adapted the approach used by McConahy and colleagues[33,34] and computed, for each child, an average portion size *z* score. Because foods have different units of measurement, the use of *z* scores standardized food portions and allowed us to incorporate foods with different units of measurement into a single variable. For an individual food, *z* scores express each portion size in terms of standard deviations from the sample mean.

Figure 1. Average portion size declines as the number of eating occasions goes up.

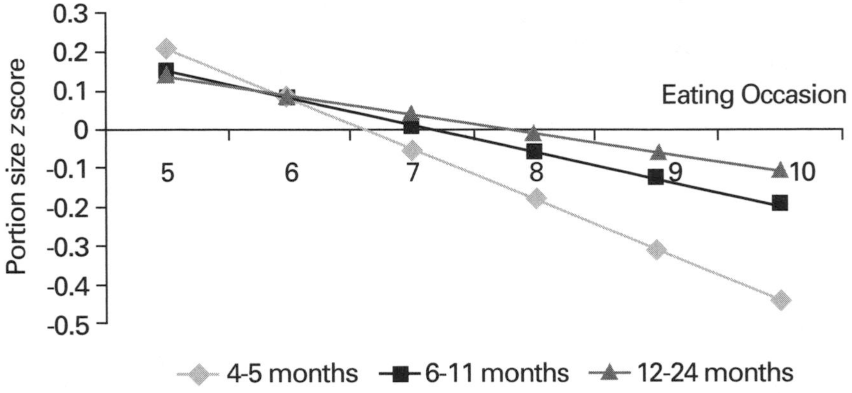

Data are from the 2002 Feeding Infants and Toddlers Study.[35] Models were adjusted for age, weight-for-age, race/ethnicity, mother's employment status, mother's education and household income. All models were significant at the *P*<.001 level.

A first set of multivariate regression models documented the fact that children's energy intakes are influenced by all of the factors thought to predict energy intake: consuming larger-than-average portions, eating more often during the day, eating more unique foods and consuming a more energy-dense diet.[35] A second set of regression models examined the relationships between: (a) portion size and the number of eating occasions, and (b) portion size and energy density. Separate models were run for 3 age groups: infants 4 to 5 months, infants 6 to 11 months and toddlers 12 to 24 months. Figure 1 summarizes the results from the model that assessed the relationship between average portion size and number of eating occasions. A significant negative association was observed, for all age groups, between the number of eating occasions and average portion size *z* scores. This indicates that, other regulation variables held constant, children who eat less often during the day consume larger-than-average portion sizes and children who eat more often during the day consume smaller-than-average portions.[35]

Figure 2. Among infants, but not toddlers, average portion size declines as energy density goes up.

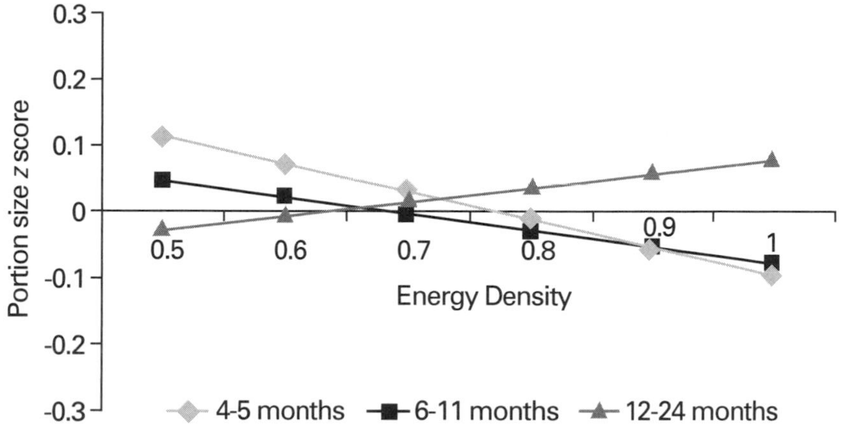

Data are from the 2002 Feeding Infants and Toddlers Study.[35] Models were adjusted for age, weight-for-age, race/ethnicity, mother's employment status, mother's education and household income. Models for both groups of infants were significant at the $P<.001$ level.

In contrast, the relationship between energy density and portion size varied across age groups.[35] As illustrated in Figure 2, a significant negative association was noted between energy density and average portion size *z* scores for both groups of infants. This indicates that, as the energy density of the diet goes down, infants consume larger-than-average portions and, as the energy density of the diet goes up, they consume smaller-than-average portions. For toddlers, however, there was no significant association between average portion size *z* scores and energy density.

These results show that infants and toddlers compensate for variation in the number of eating occasions by adjusting their portion sizes.[35] The negative association between energy density and average portion size *z* scores among infants indicates that they also compensate for changes in energy density by adjusting the amount of food consumed. The lack of a comparable association between energy density and portion size among toddlers suggests a diminished response to changes in energy density. This is consistent with findings from other research that has shown that young children's responsiveness to changes in energy density can be readily disrupted by controlling child-feeding practices that attempt to regulate what and how much children eat.[36]

These findings underscore the importance of educating parents and caregivers about the potential adverse effects that coercive feeding behaviors can have on children's innate ability to regulate energy intake. This includes not only admonitions to "clean your plate," but overrestriction of intake that may be motivated by concerns that children are overeating.[31,35] As Satter has noted, "Effective feeding demands a division of responsibility: The parent is responsible for *what* the child is offered to eat; the child is responsible for *how much* and even *whether* to eat."[37]

Infant Feeding Transitions Occur Early

Sometime during the first year of life, infants begin to consume complementary foods. There is some disagreement among experts about the preferred age at which parents and/or caregivers should introduce complementary foods.[20] Many expert groups recommend exclusive breastfeeding for the first 6 months of life,[38,39] while others recommend the introduction of appropriate solid foods when infants are developmentally ready, which is typically between 4 and 6 months after birth.[40] The American Academy of Pediatrics recommends that infants and toddlers should not be fed cow's milk before 12 months of age,[41] and juice before 6 months of age.[42]

FITS data show that many infants are fed solid foods — such as infant cereals or pureed baby foods — at early ages. About 3 out of 10 infants were introduced to solid foods before 4 months of age (see Figure 3). Only 6% of infants were 6 months or older before being introduced to solid foods.[19]

Most, but not all, parents and caregivers avoided feeding cow's milk to infants under 12 months of age and juice to infants under 6 months of age.[17,43] Infant formula was the most common source of milk in this age group, and consumption of cow's milk was rare among infants younger than 9 months of age (see Table 2). By 9 to 11 months of age, however, 20% of infants consumed cow's milk. More than 20% of infants 4 to 6 months of age consumed fruit juice.[17,43]

Figure 3. Almost 3 out of 10 infants are introduced to solid food before 4 months of age.

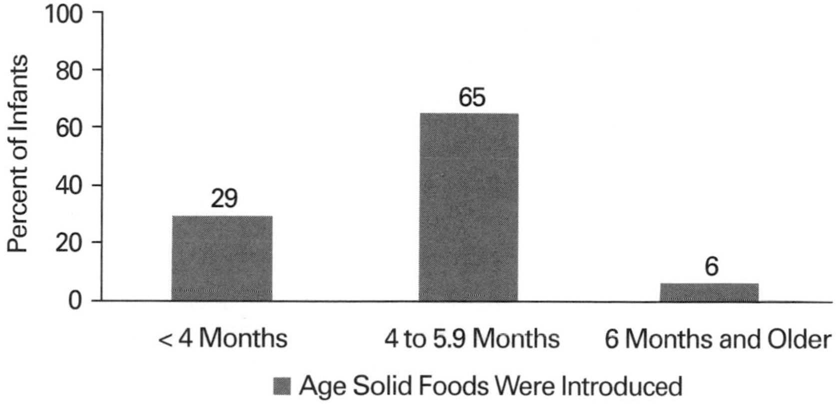

Data are from the 2002 Feeding Infants and Toddlers Study.[19] Adapted from *Journal of the American Dietetic Association,* V104, S31-S37, Briefel R, Reidy K, Karwe V, Devaney B, Feeding Infants and Toddlers Study: improvements needed in meeting infant feeding recommendations, ©2004, with permission from The American Dietetic Association.

Table 2. Percent of Infants Consuming Different Types of Milk and 100% Fruit Juice

	Percent of Infants by Age Consuming at Least Once per Day					
	4-6 mo	**7-8 mo**	**9-11 mo**	**12-14 mo**	**15-18 mo**	**19-24 mo**
Any milk	100	100	100	99	95	93
Breast milk	40	26	21	14	4	5
Formula	74	82	75	21	5	2
Cow's milk	1	3	20	85	88	88
100% juice	21	46	55	56	58	62

Data are from the 2002 Feeding Infants and Toddlers Study.[17,43]

Figure 4. Sources of food energy in the diets of infants and toddlers.

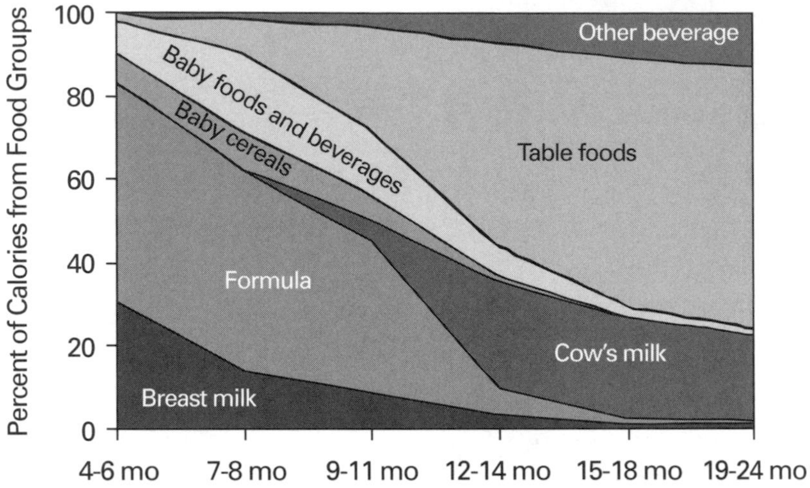

Data are from the 2002 Feeding Infants and Toddlers Study and are adapted from Fox et al.[44] Adapted from *Journal of the American Dietetic Association,* V106, S28-S42, Fox MK, Reidy K, Novak T, Ziegler P, Sources of energy and nutrients in the diets of infants and toddlers, ©2006 with permission from The American Dietetic Association

A simple and intuitive, yet very powerful, story about transitions in infant feeding emerges from an analysis of the composition of the diets of infants and toddlers (see Figure 4).

As expected, at young ages, calorie intakes are accounted for largely by breast milk and formula:

- Some 84% of the calories consumed by infants 4 to 6 months of age came from breast milk or formula
- Another 17% of their calories came from other foods, with the largest share coming from infant cereals and baby foods

For older infants, the share of calories from breast milk and formula declined, again as expected, and other food sources — especially baby foods, beverages and baby cereals — became more important.[44]

At 9 to 11 months, a *major* transition in infant feeding occurs. Infant foods — such as breast milk, formula and prepared baby foods — begin to be replaced at an increasing rate by table foods, as depicted in Figure 4. By 19 to 24 months of age, table foods account for the majority of toddlers' calories. The foods that caregivers select to provide these calories can have a profound effect on children's diets. The remainder of this chapter provides insights into the choices caregivers are making.

Infants and Toddlers Are Not Eating Fruits and Vegetables

Fruits and vegetables are a cornerstone of a healthy diet. Because food acceptance patterns form early in life, it is important for parents and caregivers to introduce older infants and toddlers to a wide variety of fruits and vegetables, and encourage their acceptance of them.[3,4,45] Specific types of vegetables — including dark green, leafy vegetables, such as broccoli, spinach and other greens, and deep yellow vegetables, such as carrots, sweet potatoes and winter squash — are especially important because they are concentrated sources of nutrients known to be lacking in the diets of young children.[20]

FITS data show that substantial proportions of infants and toddlers consumed no discrete fruits or vegetables (excluding small amounts of fruits and vegetables in mixed dishes such as pizza and spaghetti). Only 76% of infants 7 to 8 months of age consumed any type of fruit, and this proportion declined with age (see Table 3). By 19 to 24 months, 33% of toddlers did not consume any fresh, canned, jarred or frozen fruit.[17]

Trends in vegetable intake are notably different. At 7 to 8 months of age, roughly 67% of infants consumed some type of vegetable in a day. By 19 to 24 months, the proportion consuming vegetables increased to 82%.[17] However, this finding is not as positive as it may seem. It turns out that a major driver of vegetable consumption was French fries. By 15 to 18 months of age, French fries were the most commonly consumed vegetable (see Figure 5). When French fries are not included in tabulations, the prevalence of vegetable consumption was essentially flat from 9 to 24 months of age, with more than a quarter of infants and toddlers consuming no vegetables on the day that parents were questioned about consumption.[17]

Table 3. Percent of Infants and Toddlers Consuming Fruits and Vegetables

	Percent of Infants and Toddlers Consuming at Least Once per Day					
	4-6 mos	**7-8 mos**	**9-11 mos**	**12-14 mos**	**15-18 mos**	**19-24 mos**
Any Fruit	42	76	76	77	72	67
Baby Food Fruit	39	68	45	16	4	2
Types of Fruit						
Apples	19	33	32	28	20	22
Bananas	16	31	35	38	32	30
Berries	<1	<1	5	7	11	8
Citrus	<1	<1	2	5	7	5
Melons	<1	1	4	7	7	10
Any Vegetable	40	67	73	77	79	82
Baby Food Vegetables	36	55	34	13	3	2
Cooked Vegetables	5	17	46	66	73	76
Raw Vegetables	<1	2	6	8	14	19
Types of Vegetables						
Dark Green Vegetables[a]	<1	3	4	5	10	8
Deep Yellow Vegetables[b]	27	39	29	24	14	13
White Potatoes	4	12	24	33	42	41
Other Starchy Vegetables[c]	7	11	17	17	21	24

Data are from the 2002 Feeding Infants and Toddlers Study.[17]

[a]Broccoli, spinach, romaine lettuce and other greens.

[b]Carrots, pumpkin, sweet potato and winter squash.

[c]Corn, green peas, lima beans, black-eyed peas (not dried), cassava and rutabaga.

Reprinted from *Journal of the American Dietetic Association,* V104, S45-S50, Fox MK, Pac S, Devaney B, Jankowski L, Feeding Infants and Toddlers Study: what foods are infants and toddlers eating? ©2004 with permission from The American Dietetic Association

Figure 5. By 15-18 months, fried potatoes are the most commonly consumed vegetable.

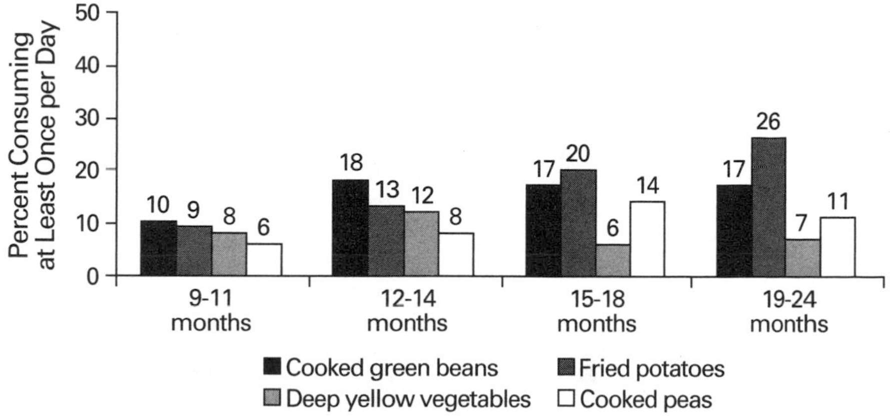

Data are from the 2002 Feeding Infants and Toddlers Study.[17] Adapted from *Journal of the American Dietetic Association,* V104, S45-S50, Fox MK, Pac S, Devaney B, Jankowski L, Feeding infants and toddlers study: what foods are infants and toddlers eating? ©2004, with permission from The American Dietetic Association.

The FITS data also indicate that consumption of nutrient-dense vegetables is low (see Table 3). For most age groups, fewer than 10% consumed dark green, leafy vegetables.[17] Consumption of deep yellow vegetables was more common, but declined substantially with age — dropping from 39% at 7 to 8 months of age to 13% at 19 to 24 months of age.[17]

Many Infants and Toddlers Consume High-Calorie, Low-Nutrient Foods

Meeting the energy and nutrient needs of toddlers leaves little room for foods that provide calories but few nutrients.[46] In fact, thoughtful selection of foods is required to meet nutrient needs without exceeding calorie requirements. The FITS data show that there is room for improvement in the choices parents and caregivers are making. Increased consumption of table foods generally is associated with higher calorie intakes and decreased intakes of 1 or more essential nutrients.[18] This is especially true for the youngest infants.

Figure 6. Substantial proportions of infants and toddlers consume sweets and salty snacks.

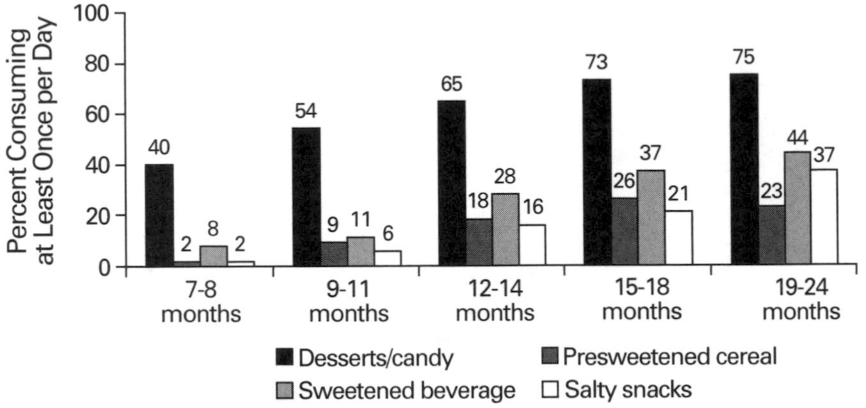

Data are from the 2002 Feeding Infants and Toddlers Study.[17] Adapted from *Journal of the American Dietetic Association,* V104, S45-S50, Fox MK, Pac S, Devaney B, Jankowski L, Feeding infants and toddlers study: what foods are infants and toddlers eating? ©2004, with permission from The American Dietetic Association.

Part of the problem is frequent consumption of desserts and candy. Among infants as young as 7 to 8 months of age, 40% consumed a dessert or candy in a given day (see Figure 6).[17] Among toddlers 19 to 24 months of age, this percentage increased to 75%. In fact, by 15 to 18 months of age, more toddlers consumed desserts and candy than consumed fruit (see Table 3 and Figure 6).

Salty snacks, such as potato chips, also appear in the diet at an early age. At 12 to 14 months of age, 16% of children consumed salty snacks in a day; by 19 to 24 months, more than one quarter of toddlers consumed salty snacks.[17]

Presweetened cereals and sweetened beverages also are prevalent in the diets of toddlers. By 19 to 24 months of age, 44% of toddlers consumed sweetened beverages. These beverages were most often fruit-flavored drinks (38%), but more than 10% of children in this age group consumed carbonated soda.[17] While juices that are 100% fruit juice can be a source of some nutrients, primarily vitamin C, overreliance on juice can replace other nutritious foods and lead to excess calorie intake. For this reason, the American Academy of

Pediatrics recommends that juice intake be limited to 4 to 6 fluid ounces per day, and that whole fruits rather than juices be used to provide the recommended daily fruit servings.[42] An Institute of Medicine committee recently proposed that WIC food packages for children be revised to incorporate this recommendation.[20] FITS data indicate that, for most age groups, more than 50% of all children consume juice in a day. For children under 15 months of age, the average amount consumed per day falls within the recommended range of 4 to 6 fluid ounces. Among children 15 to 24 months of age, however, the average amount of juice consumed — 9 to 10 fluid ounces — is substantially greater than recommended.[43]

Discussion

FITS has made an important contribution to our knowledge about the dietary intake of infants and toddlers. It is the first national study with sample sizes large enough to support detailed analysis of dietary intake in narrowly defined age groups of children under 2 years of age. Analysis of FITS data showed that, overall, the diets of infants and toddlers in the United States are nutritionally adequate. However, infants and toddlers appear to be consuming too many calories. Children's natural ability to self-regulate energy intake appears to be diminishing at early ages (before the age of 2). The imposition of controlling feeding practices is one factor that may contribute to this problem.

There also are noteworthy problems with the food choices some parents and caregivers are making for their children. Many parents and caregivers are introducing infants to solid foods, cow's milk and juices too early. In addition, the diets of infants and toddlers exhibit problematic patterns. These patterns are reflective of the family diet, or the "typical American diet," with its well-established nutritional shortcomings, which infants and toddlers gradually adopt. In children under 2 years of age, we see a diet that lacks fruits and vegetables, especially nutrient-dense vegetables, frequent consumption of foods that are high in added sugars, consumption of salty snacks and excess consumption of juices. Some of these eating patterns emerge at surprisingly early ages.

A main message from FITS is that pediatric healthcare professionals need to encourage parents and caregivers to think about the quality of the foods they are feeding their children, as well as when to introduce specific kinds of foods.

It is important to emphasize that food preferences are established early in life and may predict future eating habits. Healthy eating habits should begin to be formed at birth — with breastfeeding — and continue through infancy, guided by recommended infant feeding practices. Once solid foods have been introduced, fruits and vegetables, along with whole grains, should form the cornerstone of a healthy diet. Older infants and toddlers should consume several different types of fruit and vegetables each day, in an array of colors. (The more colorful a fruit or vegetable is, the more nutrients it provides.) Desserts, candy, sweetened beverages and salty snacks should be offered infrequently. Nutrient-dense, age-appropriate snacks such as fruit, whole grain crackers and cereals, cheese and yogurt should be emphasized in the diet. Juice consumption should be limited to 4 to 6 fluid ounces per day. Formula or milk should be offered at mealtimes, and water is the preferred thirst quencher.

Acknowledgments

The authors wish to acknowledge the following colleagues who were coauthors on 1 or more of the papers summarized here: Ronette Briefel, Paula Ziegler, Susan Pac, Kathleen Reidy, Michael Ponza, Susan Barr, Kristy Hendricks, Jean Skinner, Tim Novak, Vatsala Karwe, Carol Razafindrakoto and Linda Jankowski.

References

1. Birch LL. The role of experience in children's food acceptance patterns. *Journal of the American Dietetic Association.* 1987;87:S36-S40.
2. Birch LL. Development of food acceptance patterns in the first years of life. *Proceedings of the Nutrition Society.* 1998;57:617-624.
3. Mennella J, Beauchamp GK. Early flavor experiences: research update. *Nutrition Reviews.* 1998; 56:205-211.
4. Krebs-Smith SM, Heimendinger J, Patterson BH, et al. Psychological factors associated with fruit and vegetable consumption. *American Journal of Health Promotion.* 1995;10:98-104.
5. Birch LL, Fisher JO. Appetite and eating behavior in children. *Pediatric Clinics of North America.* 1995;42:931-953.
6. Birch LL, McPhee L, Shoba BC, Steinberg L, Krehbiel R. Clean up your plate: effects of child feeding practices on the condition of meal size. *Learning Motivation.* 1987;18:301-317.
7. Bergmann KE, Bergmann RL, Von Kries R. Early determinants of childhood overweight and adiposity in a birth cohort study: role of breastfeeding. *International Journal of Obesity-Related Metabolic Disorders.* 2003;27:162-172.
8. Devaney B, Kalb L, Briefel R, Zavitsky-Novak T, Clusen N, Ziegler P. Feeding Infants and Toddlers Study: overview of the study design. *Journal of the American Dietetic Association.* 2004;104:S8-S13.

9. Ziegler P, Briefel R, Clusen N, Devaney B. Feeding Infants and Toddlers Study (FITS): development of the FITS survey in comparison to other survey methods. *Journal of the American Dietetic Association.* 2006;106:S12-S27.
10. Institute of Medicine. Food and Nutrition Board. *Dietary Reference Intakes: Calcium, Phosphorus, Magnesium, Vitamin D, Fluoride.* Washington, DC: National Academy Press; 1999.
11. Institute of Medicine. Food and Nutrition Board. *Dietary Reference Intakes for Vitamin C, Vitamin E, Selenium, and Carotenoids.* Washington, DC: National Academy Press; 2000.
12. Institute of Medicine. Food and Nutrition Board. *Dietary Reference Intakes for Thiamin, Riboflavin, Niacin, Vitamin B6, Folate, Vitamin B12, Pantothenic Acid, Biotin, and Choline.* Washington, DC: National Academy Press; 2000.
13. Institute of Medicine. Food and Nutrition Board. *Dietary Reference Intakes: Vitamin A, Vitamin K, Arsenic, Boron, Chromium, Copper, Iodine, Iron, Manganese, Molybdenum, Nickel, Silicon, Valadium, and Zinc.* Washington, DC: National Academy Press; 2002.
14. Institute of Medicine. Food and Nutrition Board. *Dietary Reference Intakes: Energy, Carbohydrate, Fiber, Fat, Fatty Acids, Cholesterol, Protein, and Amino Acids.* Washington, DC: National Academy Press; 2002.
15. Institute of Medicine. Food and Nutrition Board. *Dietary Reference Intakes for Water, Potassium, Sodium, Chloride, and Sulfate.* Washington, DC: National Academy Press; 2004.
16. Devaney B, Ziegler P, Pac S, Karwe V, Barr SI. Nutrient intakes of infants and toddlers. *Journal of the American Dietetic Association.* 2004;104:S14-S21.
17. Fox MK, Pac S, Devaney B, Jankowski L. Feeding Infants and Toddlers Study: what foods are infants and toddlers eating? *Journal of the American Dietetic Association.* 2004;104:S22-S30.
18. Briefel R, Reidy K, Karwe V, Jankowski L, Hendricks K. Toddlers' transition to table foods: impact on nutrient intakes and food patterns. *Journal of the American Dietetic Association.* 2004;104: S38-S44.
19. Briefel R, Reidy K, Karwe V, Devaney B. Feeding Infants and Toddlers Study: improvements needed in meeting infant feeding recommendations. *Journal of the American Dietetic Association.* 2004; 104:S31-S37.
20. Institute of Medicine, Committee to Review the WIC Food Packages. Food and Nutrition Board. *WIC Food Packages: Time for a Change.* Washington, DC: National Academy Press; 2005.
21. Devaney B, Kim M, Carriquiry A, Camaño-Garcia G. *Assessing the Nutrient Intakes of Vulnerable Subgroups.* US Department of Agriculture, Economic Research Service. Contractor and Cooperator Report No. 11, 2005. Available at: http://www.ers.usda.gov. Accessed November 15, 2005.
22. Fox MK, Cole N. *Nutrition and Health Characteristics of Low-Income Populations, Volume I: Food Stamp Participants and Non-participants.* US Department of Agriculture, Economic Research Service, Electronic publication number E-FAN-04-010-1, 2004. Available at: http://www.ers.usda.gov. Accessed June 16, 2005.
23. *Continuing Survey of Food Intakes by Individuals 1994-96* [book on CD-ROM]. Beltsville, Md: US Department of Agriculture, Agricultural Research Service; 1998.
24. Young LR, Nestle M. The contribution of expanding portion sizes to the US obesity epidemic. *American Journal of Public Health.* 2002;92:246-249.
25. Hill JO, Peters JC. Environmental contributions to the obesity epidemic. *Science.* 1998;280: 1371-1374.
26. Rolls BJ, Engell D, Birch LL. Serving portion size influences 5-year-old but not 3-year-old children's food intakes. *Journal of the American Dietetic Association.* 2000;100:232-234.
27. Shea S, Basch CE, Contento IR, Zybert P. Variability and self-regulation of energy intake in young children in their everyday environment. *Pediatrics.* 1992;90:542-546.
28. Birch LL, Fisher JO. Development of eating behaviors among children and adolescents. *Pediatrics.* 1998;101:539-549.
29. Adair LS. The infant's ability to self-regulate caloric intake: a case study. *Journal of the American Dietetic Association.* 1984;84:543-546.

30. Dewey KG. Nutrition, growth, and complementary feeding of the breastfed infant. *Pediatric Clinics of North America.* 2001;48:87-104.
31. Birch LL, Davison KK. Family environmental factors influencing the developing behavioral controls of food intake and childhood overweight. *Pediatric Clinics of North America.* 2001;48:893-907.
32. Wilson JF. Preschool children maintain intake of other foods at a meal including sugared chocolate milk. *Appetite.* 2000;16:61-67.
33. McConahy MS, Smiciklas-Wright H, Birch LL, Mitchell DC, Picciano MF. Food portions are positively related to energy intake and body weight in early childhood. *Journal of Pediatrics.* 2002; 140:340-347.
34. McConahy KL, Smiciklas-Wright H, Mitchell DC, Picciano MF. Portion size of common foods predicts energy intake among preschool-aged children. *Journal of the American Dietetic Association.* 2004;104:975-979.
35. Fox MK, Devaney B, Reidy K, Razafindrakoto C, Ziegler P. Relationship between portion size and energy intake among infants and toddlers: evidence of self-regulation. *Journal of the American Dietetic Association.* 2006;106:S77-S81.
36. Birch LL, McPhee L, Shoba BC, Steinberg L, Krehbiel R. "Clean up your plate": effects of child feeding practices on the condition of meal size. *Learning and Motivation.* 1987;18:301-317.
37. Satter E. Comments from a practitioner on Leann Birch's research. *Journal of the American Dietetic Association.* 1987;87:S41-S43.
38. American Academy of Pediatrics, Section on Breastfeeding. Breastfeeding and the use of human milk. *Pediatrics.* 2005;115:496-506.
39. World Health Organization. *The Optimal Duration of Exclusive Breastfeeding: Report of an Expert Consultation.* Geneva, Switzerland: World Health Organization; 2001.
40. American Academy of Pediatrics. Complementary feeding. In: *Pediatric Nutrition Handbook.* 5th ed. Elk Grove Village, Ill: American Academy of Pediatrics; 2004:103-109.
41. American Academy of Pediatrics, Committee on Nutrition. The use of whole cow's milk in infancy. *Pediatrics.* 1992;89:1105-1109.
42. American Academy of Pediatrics, Committee on Nutrition. The use and misuse of fruit juice in pediatrics. *Pediatrics.* 2001;107:1210-1213.
43. Skinner J, Ziegler P, Ponza M. Transitions in infants' and toddlers' beverage patterns. *Journal of the American Dietetic Association.* 2004;104:S45-S50.
44. Fox MK, Reidy K, Novak T, Ziegler P. Sources of energy and nutrients in the diets of infants and toddlers. *Journal of the American Dietetic Association.* 2006;106:S28-S42.
45. World Health Organization. *Infant and Young Child Nutrition. Global Strategy for Infant and Young Child Feeding.* Report by the Secretariat. Document EB109/12. Geneva, Switzerland: World Health Organization; 2001.
46. Butte N, Cobb K, Dwyer J, Graney L, Heird W, Rickard K. The Start Healthy Feeding Guidelines for infants and toddlers. *Journal of the American Dietetic Association.* 2004;104:442-454.

Feeding Children in an Environment of Plenty: Lessons From the Laboratory

Jennifer Orlet Fisher, PhD
Leann L. Birch, PhD

Introduction

For most of human history, children have eaten in conditions of scarcity, with much of family life devoted to the procurement and preparation of food. In sharp contrast, today in non-Third World countries children's eating habits tend to develop under unprecedented conditions of dietary abundance: Food and drink are available in most venues of everyday life — from the home, school, restaurant and grocery store to the library, mall, community center and every convenience store in between.

As of 2004, there were 528,940 food-service establishments in the United States and an additional 152,521 stores where food and beverages could be purchased.[1] In addition, a growing variety of inexpensive and energy-dense foods have become available in larger and larger portions: For example, a typical American supermarket carries 45,000 items today[2] — and consumer portions served by restaurants and fast-food establishments are often double the size currently recommended.[3] Researchers who have witnessed rapid increases in the prevalence of overweight among American children and children in other developed countries have focused their attention on understanding how the environment in which children eat contributes to the problem.

This chapter will review research indicating that young children are exposed to conditions of dietary excess through the ecology of the family eating environment.

The New Family Table: Less Time, More Food

In the home, most women still hold the primary responsibility for feeding children.[4] Changes in employment and family composition, however, suggest that women have less time to devote to this activity. From 1975 to 2004, labor force participation among mothers with children under 18 years of age increased from 47% to 71%.[5] In 61% of 2-parent families with children under 18 years of age, both parents work.[6] Among single mothers, 72% are employed.[6] Additionally, more women than men parent and feed their children without the assistance of a spouse: 19% of children under 18 years of age live with their mother only.[7]

One consequence of these trends is that young children are routinely fed by someone other than a parent: In fact, 30% of preschool-age children receive childcare — which includes mealtime care — from a grandparent or other relative, and 23% participate in organized childcare.[8] In addition, families spend less time eating meals together: As many as 8% to 16% of married parents and 11% to 22% of single parents eat dinner with their preschool-age child 2 days each week or less.[9] Finally, less of the food that children eat is prepared at home and served at the family table.[10] More than 2 out of every 5 family food dollars is now spent on food away from the home,[11] where children may be served particularly large portions[12] and consume more energy and fat than when eating at home.[13]

Collectively, these circumstances mean that children are eating at an increasing distance from the hands that have traditionally fed them — which affects the ingredients and preparation of the foods they consume, as well as the social influences surrounding their eating.

Parenting in an Environment of Plenty

How do parents approach feeding their children? Parenting is driven largely by what parents want for their children and parents' perceptions of the environmental threats to attaining those goals.[14] The most basic goals of feeding children are universal: All parents want for their children survival and healthy growth and development. However, the specific strategies that parents use to feed their children are dictated by the cultural and contextual interpretations of those goals, as well as the actual and perceived threats to their attainment.

Historically, limited food resources have posed a major threat to the health and well-being of children.[15] For as long as these conditions prevailed, parenting strategies to feed children were handed down from one generation to the next and were a traditional part of nurturing children — and a large, robust child was testament to the effectiveness of those efforts.

Although parents' universal goals for their children's growth and health remain unchanged, the food environment has changed dramatically in recent decades. The increasing presence of overweight children in the United States and other developed countries suggests that limited food resources are no longer a pressing threat to child health. Traditional feeding concerns and strategies — that developed in response to food scarcity — may be ineffective or even counterproductive under conditions of plenty.

Are Healthy Eaters Born or Made?

> *The taste decides; the teeth are put in action, the tongue unites with the palate in tasting, and the stomach soon commences the process of assimilation.*[15]
> — Jean Anthelme Brillat-Savarin

Taste predispositions are believed to form the basis of food acceptance and preference patterns in early development. (For more information, see the chapter in this text by Julie Mennella.) Innate predispositions to prefer sweet tastes and reject tastes that are bitter are postulated to have evolved as protective measures that encourage the ingestion of energy-rich foods and prevent the ingestion of toxic substances, particularly in early development. In fact, children learn to prefer flavors that are associated with foods containing high amounts of energy.[16] Even preferences for foods not considered to be energy-dense, such as vegetables, are tied to energy content: Those fruits and vegetables with higher energy content, such as potatoes and bananas, are preferred over those foods with less energy content, such as lettuce and cabbage.[17]

Humans have evolved to prefer foods that provide adequate energy, and to consume those foods in sufficient quantities to survive. The question of whether children can self-regulate energy intake is not new. Clara Davis conducted seminal research in the late 1920s and 1930s, providing the first evidence of an unlearned ability to self-regulate energy intake in infancy.[18,19]

In the studies undertaken by Davis, infants and toddlers grew well and had few illnesses when given the opportunity to select and consume a variety of simply prepared foods at each meal.[18,19] Almost a half century later, Fomon and colleagues revisited the issue of self-regulation of energy intake by systematically varying the energy density of infant formula.[20,21] By 6 weeks of age, full-term infants who were fed a concentrated formula (100 kcal/mL) consumed smaller volumes than did those infants who were fed a diluted formula (54 kcal/mL), such that total daily energy intake did not differ between the 2 groups. In 1977, observational data from Pearcey and de Castro complemented these experimental findings, revealing that individual variability in energy consumed at meals among 12-month-old infants was close to 47%, while variability in daily energy intake was 17%.[22] Similarly, Cohen and colleagues found no difference in daily energy intake among infants 4 to 6 months of age who were fed only breast milk versus those who were fed breast milk along with complementary foods.[23]

The ability to regulate energy intake has also been described in preschool-age children.[24-28] Children responded to covert manipulations in the energy content of foods served as a first course by adjusting their subsequent intake, such that their total energy intake for the meal[24,25] and energy consumed over a 30-hour period[26] were maintained across conditions in which low- or high-energy foods were provided as a first course. Differences among preschool-age children in their ability to self-regulate energy intake have been associated with differences in weight status.[27,28]

The regulation of energy intake in early development may be viewed as an unlearned ability as well as the opportunity to exercise this control.[29] That children are capable of self-regulating energy intake under laboratory conditions, in the absence of adult intervention, does not speak to the extent to which this ability is exercised in the family environment.

Lessons on Eating From the Laboratory: Parents as Providers, Models and Teachers

Several decades of research inside and outside of the laboratory reveal the strong influence that caregivers have on children's eating through selecting the foods that make up the family diet, serving as models of eating that children learn to emulate, and using feeding practices to socialize eating behavior.

Adults as Providers

Children learn to like what is familiar to them. After just one exposure to a new food, intake of that food as well as similar foods by infants 4 months of age to 6 months of age nearly doubled.[30] In another study, infants who were breastfed showed the greatest increases in their intake of the first vegetable presented to them with repeated exposure to that vegetable.[31] Children exposed to a sweet, salty or plain version of a novel food showed increasing preference for the version that became familiar after being served 15 times and decreasing preference for the other versions.[32]

In a home-based intervention to increase preschool-age children's liking for a previously disliked vegetable, providing parents with nutritional advice and information did not affect children's behavior; however, giving children a taste of the vegetable over a 2-week period produced significant increases in their preference for and intake of the food.[33]

Observational studies have produced similar findings. The extent to which fruits and vegetables are present in the home and in a form and location that is conducive to consumption is correlated positively with the level of consumption in school-age children.[34-36] Accessibility appears to be particularly important for children with low preferences for fruit, 100% fruit juice and vegetables.[36] The findings are much the same for milk drinking: In a study of beverage intake among girls during middle childhood, milk consumption among girls who were almost always or always served milk at meals and snacks was 2 times higher than it was for girls who were served milk rarely or never.[37] Similarities in milk intake among mothers and daughters were also attributable to the extent that milk was served at meals.

Children's intake of particular foods is influenced not only by the types of foods present in the home but also by the amount of those foods that is available to them. Recent laboratory studies (as well as unpublished data provided by the authors and Rolls, January 2005) provide causal evidence that large food portions promote greater energy intake by children as young as 2 years of age.[38-39] When age-appropriate portions of an entrée were doubled in size, preschool-age children ate approximately 25% to 29% more than the age-appropriate portions of those foods, even though they consumed only two thirds of the smaller portions of the entrée and were not aware of increases in the portion size[39] (also JO Fisher, unpublished data, January 2005). These effects were attributable principally to increases in the average size of children's bites. Children did not adequately reduce their intake of other foods to compensate for their intake of larger portions of the entrée. As a result, energy intake was 9% to 15% higher at meals during which larger portions were served.

Adults, like children, eat more when served large portions.[40-45] In the study undertaken by the authors and Rolls (unpublished data, April 2006) of 59 low-income Hispanic and black families, total daily intake of food by family members was 6% to 9% greater when large portions of an entrée were served at successive meals. In an earlier study, Rolls and colleagues reported that adult men and women consumed 30% more energy when served a portion of macaroni and cheese that was twice the size of the smallest portion (500 g) served to a control group.[46] For both children and adults, the intake of large portions is not associated with weight status, suggesting that the relevance of large portions to weight gain is a function of exposure to large portions, rather than a particular susceptibility of the overweight individual to overeat. Evidence from laboratory studies suggests that larger portions served to consumers by restaurants, in convenience and grocery stores, and in other retail settings are driving increases in the average size of portions consumed both in and away from home,[12] as well as increases of the daily energy intake of children.[47,48]

Adults as Models

Children learn about food through the direct experience of eating and by observing the eating behavior of others. Birch found that the selection and consumption of vegetables by preschool-age children were influenced more by the choices of their peers than by their own actual preferences.[49] When preschool-age children observed the eating behavior of adults, it had a similar effect: Hendy and Raudenbush found that children's intake of a novel food increased at those meals during which they observed a teacher enthusiastically consuming the food.[50] Interestingly, enthusiastic modeling by a teacher was not as effective when children were seated with peers who exhibited different food preferences than did their teachers.[51] While one might expect modeling by parents to have a similar if not stronger influence on children's preference and choices, experimental evidence is lacking.

Studies conducted outside the laboratory also provide evidence of the role of social modeling. For example, low-income adolescent girls who reported seeing their fathers consume milk had higher calcium intakes than did those girls who did not see their fathers drink milk.[52] Parental modeling has also been associated with greater fruit juice and vegetable intake among school-age children.[53,54]

Parents as Teachers

Parents directly interact with their children during mealtimes and other eating times in a manner that facilitates the acquisition of the eating rules and norms of their particular family and culture. The degree to which children are provided autonomy in eating is one aspect of the parent–child feeding interaction that has relevance for fostering or hindering healthy eating and growth. Highly controlling approaches to feeding have unintended effects on children's food preferences and their self-regulation of energy intake. In laboratory studies of eating styles it was also concluded that higher levels of control in feeding are associated with poorer self-regulation of energy intake in preschool-age children.[27] However, the manner in which eating behavior is affected depends on the nature of the directive: For example, using food as a reward increased preschool-age children's preferences for those foods,[55] whereas requiring children to consume particular foods in order to obtain a reward ultimately engendered dislike for those foods.[56,57] Cross-sectional studies have reported that higher levels of parental control and pressure to eat were associated with lower fruit and vegetable intake[58-60] and higher intake of dietary fat[61] among young girls.

Excessive parental control and pressure to eat appear to disrupt children's short-term behavioral control of food intake. For example, in a study of children's feeding practices, it was found that encouraging children to eat by focusing their attention on the amount of food on the plate promotes greater consumption and makes children less sensitive to the caloric content of the foods consumed.[62] Likewise, Fisher and Birch found that restricting children's access to a preferred food resulted in increased selection and intake of that food when they were allowed to freely consume it.[63] Research with animal models that varied the access that nonenergy-deprived rats had to a preferred food source obtained similar findings.[64]

Food Intake and Weight

Given that pressure to eat often results in eating beyond satiation and restrictions on eating also promote overeating, one would expect to see a positive correlation between a child's energy intake and his/her body weight. However, observational studies have provided mixed support for this relationship. In middle-income, non-Hispanic white families, higher levels of restriction predicted greater eating in the absence of hunger and weight gain during middle childhood among girls, particularly among those who were initially overweight or who had an overweight mother.[65,66] In another prospective study, parental restrictions on eating among children 5 years of age predicted higher body mass index (BMI) *z* scores at 7 years of age among both boys and girls with overweight mothers.[67] Conversely, higher levels of pressure to eat have been associated with lower total body fat in African-American and white boys and girls,[68] as well as reduced BMI *z* scores in children between 5 years of age and 7 years of age who had overweight mothers.[67] In contrast, in other research, parental control of feeding was not associated with either children's eating behavior or their weight.[69,70] The reason for these inconsistencies is unclear.

Systematic investigation of environmental influences on children's eating behavior and weight is *still* in its infancy, and scientific understanding of the factors that drive weight gain and eating behavior are therefore only preliminary. Much of what is known about children and feeding comes from carefully controlled studies conducted in the laboratory. This type of research has played a critical role in evaluating *causality* in phenomena-based research. However, there is a paucity of hypothesis-driven observational research that seeks to understand the actual *context* in which eating behavior occurs.

Differing Perceptions of Healthy Weight: The Importance of Socioeconomic and Cultural Contexts

The strategies parents use to feed their children reflect their socioeconomic and cultural goals for their children's eating and health. For example, among middle-income, non-Hispanic white families, maternal perceptions of and concerns about overweight daughters were positively correlated with the use of restrictive feeding practices.[71] However, overweight is not universally perceived as a detriment to health, especially for infants and very young children.

For example, low-income mothers have reported that a heavy infant is viewed as a sign of a healthy child and successful parenting.[72] Given such values, caregivers may interpret infant behavior in terms of potential hunger and take specific care to prevent that state. Indeed, low-income mothers often interpret nonspecific behaviors, such as frequent crying and reaching towards food, as signs of hunger.[72,73] Consequently, feeding practices that are at odds with current recommendations — including concentrating formula[73] or adding cereal to it and/or introducing solid foods before 4 months of age[72-75] — may be adopted by mothers who value having bigger babies.

Cultural, socioeconomic and psychological factors also may shape parents' perceptions of a healthy weight for their children. Nationally representative data indicate that nearly one third of mothers with overweight children do not perceive their children as being overweight.[76] Among low-income populations, 70% to 80% of mothers perceive their overweight child to be of normal weight or even underweight.[77,78] In addition, low-income mothers of young children have reported that social stigmatization, physical limitations and lack of a healthy diet are more relevant indicators of problematic weight than are objective measurements.[73] These findings suggest that low-income parents desire their children to be at a healthy weight, but differ from healthcare professionals in their view of just what that "healthy" weight is.

Thus, the strategies parents use to feed their children and the effects of those strategies on children's eating and health are informed by the broader context in which feeding is embedded. The fact that feeding is influenced by culture and context does not preclude the emergence of common feeding themes that cross cultural and socioeconomic boundaries. For example, social modeling influences on eating are evident cross-culturally. Recent experimental findings have demonstrated the effects that large portions of food had on energy intake in samples of low- and middle-income Hispanic, black and white preschool-age children (Fisher, Birch, Rolls, unpublished data, July 2004). Research on restrictive feeding practices also reveals similar effects on eating behavior for low-income Hispanic and middle-income white families. Data from 320 Hispanic mothers and their children 5 to 18 years of age (n = 1038) revealed that higher levels of maternal restriction in feeding were associated with greater negative self-evaluation of eating and secretive eating among their children.[79]

Conclusions

This perspective holds that feeding is not universal in form and intent, and that the failure to take into account the goals and values that drive feeding strategies and practices may obscure the impact that those strategies and practices have on children's health. For example, an observational study by Musher-Eizenman and Holub revealed that food restrictions that were fueled by parental concerns about the child's weight increased children's externally motivated snacking, whereas restrictions prompted by a more general concern for the child's nutritional well-being were not.[80] Although the study sample was relatively homogeneous, the findings suggest that the effects of a given feeding practice on children's eating may not be clear unless the impetus for its use is understood. Research is desperately needed to understand how the meanings and intent of feeding strategies differ within and between cultures.

Implications for Practice

The growing problem of overweight among children in developed countries suggests that the current dietary environment poses a threat to the health and development of children that has not been seen in previous generations. Environmental influences on children's eating practices and their weight are filtered through the local ecology of the family. Children's food preferences and their diets reflect the foods that are available and accessible to them in part because familiarity drives preference.

The natural tendency of children to prefer energy-rich foods over energy-poor but micronutrient-rich alternatives highlights the need for adult intervention to provide a varied and healthful diet. As such, caregivers play a critical role in determining which kinds of foods will become familiar to their children — from the foods kept routinely in the cupboard to those served regularly at the family table and even those consumed away from home.

Caregivers also act as important gatekeepers to the social influences surrounding children's eating. Because observing the eating behavior of others influences children's acceptance of foods, decisions about how often families eat together and who is present during meals dictate what is consumed and what becomes preferred. Accordingly, caregivers should try to eat what they would like their children to eat, sharing not only meals but also foods. In other words, caregivers should avoid "short-order cooking." Exposing children to healthful foods in a noncoercive manner is central to engendering preference. By facilitating acceptance, repeated exposure to healthy foods and modeling healthy eating may reduce conflicts over eating.

Children possess an innate ability to self-regulate their energy intake, but the extent to which they exercise this ability is determined by the conditions of the environments in which they eat. Large food portions, highly controlling feeding practices and social examples of excessive consumption do not appear to support self-regulation of energy intake in children. Feeding strategies that are responsive to children and directly encourage their attention to hunger and fullness support self-regulation.[81] For example, children appear to serve themselves less and eat less when they are allowed to select their own portion size than when they are served large portions of food.[39]

The observation that high levels of control in feeding are counterproductive does not imply that a lack of structure in feeding is necessarily beneficial. On the contrary, it seems reasonable to expect that uninvolved and indulgent approaches to feeding promote excessive food intake and weight gain in food environments of plenty. However, there are very few empirical data available that speak to this issue. A study of 231 parents of Hispanic and black pre-school-aged children revealed that children with indulgent parents had higher body mass index *z* scores compared to children with authoritarian parents.[82] Feeding practices that provide a structure and set limits are believed to support self-regulation of energy intake, but empirical evidence for this is lacking as well.

Culture, tradition and context reveal what is valued and what actions are taken to achieve parenting goals. Feeding practices that emerged to protect children in times of scarcity are ineffective and even counterproductive in the current climate of dietary excess in the developed countries. If we, as those involved in the science of nutrition, can help parents and other caregivers understand that there are new threats to the healthy development of children in an environment of dietary excess, and can show them how alternative feeding strategies can help them address these threats, we may be able to effect change in these counterproductive practices. However, gravitation toward the use of familiar and comfortable feeding practices, without conscious thought for their impact, may pose a significant challenge for even the most motivated parents and other caregivers. Therefore, efforts to promote adaptive feeding practices in the current environment will require more than simply providing parents and caregivers with new strategies: They *must* be aware of the current threat to their children's healthy growth and development posed by the contemporary food environment, and choose to adopt feeding strategies that deal effectively with this threat.

Research in this arena will be critical to the development and dissemination of effective guidance that is specific to parents' socioeconomic backgrounds and cultures. Tailored guidance will ensure that nutritional messages motivate rather than alienate families who could greatly benefit from such assistance, but who may not have the resources to identify or implement such changes.

References

1. U.S. Census Bureau. County business patterns for the United States 2004. Table 1. Available at: http://www. census.gov/prod/2006pubs/04cbp/cb0400a1us.pdf. Accessed July 6, 2006.
2. Food Marketing Institute. Supermarket facts: industry overview 2005. Available at: http://www. fmi.org/facts_figs/superfact.htm. Accessed July 6, 2006.
3. Young LR, Nestle M. Expanding portion sizes in the US marketplace: implications for nutrition counseling. *Journal of the American Dietetic Association.* 2003;103:231-234.
4. U.S. Dept of Agriculture. Agricultural Research Service: Food Surveys Research Group. Results from USDA's 1994-96 Diet and Health Knowledge Survey: Table 11. Available at: http://www. ars.usda.gov/SP2UserFiles/Place/12355000/pdf/dhks9496.pdf. Accessed September 15, 2005.
5. U.S. Dept of Labor. Bureau of Labor Statistics. Women in the labor force: a databook. Report 985. Table 7: Employment status of women by presence and age of youngest child, 1975-2004. Available at: http://www.bls.gov/cps/wlf-databook2005.htm. Accessed September 15, 2005.
6. U.S. Dept of Labor. Bureau of Labor Statistics. Employment characteristics of families. Table 4. Families with own children: employment status of parents by age of youngest child and family type, 2004-05 annual averages. Available at: http://www.bls.gov/news.release/famee.t04.htm. Accessed July 6, 2006.
7. U.S. Census Bureau. America's families and living arrangements 2005. Table C2. Household relationship and living arrangements of children under 18 years, by age, sex, race, Hispanic origin: 2005. Available at: http://www.census.gov/population/socdemo/hh-fam/cps2005/tabC2-all.csv. Accessed July 6, 2006.
8. U.S. Census Bureau. Survey of income and program participation: who's minding the kids? Child care arrangements. Table 1. Preschoolers in types of child care arrangements: Winter 2002. Available at: http://www.census.gov.prod.2005pubs/p70-101.pdf. Accessed July 6, 2006.
9. Lugaila TA. Current population reports. A child's day: 2000. Table 2. Selected indicators of daily interaction of children under 18 with designated parent or father/stepfather if present by marital status of designated parent. [U.S. Census Bureau Web site]. Available at: http://www.sipp.census.gov/sipp/ p70s/p70-89.pdf. Accessed September 15, 2005.
10. Nielsen SJ, Siega-Riz AM, Popkin BM. Trends in energy intake in U.S. between 1977 and 1996: similar shifts seen across age groups. *Obesity Research.* 2002;10:370-378.
11. U.S. Dept of Labor. Consumer expenditures in 2004. Table A. Average annual expenditures of all consumer units and percent changes, Consumer Expenditure Survey, 2002-2004. Available at http://www.bls.gov.cx.csxann04.pdf. Accessed July 6, 2006.

12. Nielsen SJ, Popkin BM. Patterns and trends in food portion sizes, 1977-1998. *Journal of the American Medical Association.* 2003;289:450-453.
13. Bowman SA, Gortmaker SL, Ebbeling CB, Pereira MA, Ludwig DS. Effects of fast-food consumption on energy intake and diet quality among children in a national household survey. *Pediatrics.* 2004;113(1; pt 1):112-118.
14. Levine RA. Human parental care: universal goals, cultural strategies, individual behavior. In: Levine RA, Miller PM, West MM, eds. *Parental Behavior in Diverse Societies.* San Francisco, Calif: Jossey-Bass; 1988:3-12. New Directions for Child Development, No. 40: Social and Behavior Science Series.
15. Caballero B. A nutrition paradox — underweight and obesity in developing countries. *New England Journal of Medicine.* 2005;352:1514-1516.
16. Kern DL, McPhee L, Fisher J, Johnson S, Birch LL. The postingestive consequences of fat condition preferences for flavors associated with high dietary fat. *Physiology & Behavior.* 1993;54:71-76.
17. Gibson EL, Wardle J. Energy density predicts preferences for fruit and vegetables in 4-year-old children. *Appetite.* 2003;41:97-98.
18. Davis CM. Results of the self-selection of diets by young children. *The Canadian Medical Association Journal.* 1939;41:257-261.
19. Davis CM. Self-selection of diet by newly weaned infants. *American Journal of Diseases of Children.* 1928;36:651-679.
20. Fomon SJ, Filer LJ Jr, Thomas LN, Rogers RR, Proksch AM. Relationship between formula concentration and rate of growth of normal infants. *The Journal of Nutrition.* 1969;98:241-254.
21. Fomon SJ, Filmer LJ Jr, Thomas LN, Anderson TA, Nelson SE. Influence of formula concentration on caloric intake and growth of normal infants. *Acta Paediatrica Scandinavica.* 1975;64:172-181.
22. Pearcey SM, de Castro JM. Food intake and meal patterns of one year old infants. *Appetite.* 1997;29:201-212.
23. Cohen RJ, Brown KH, Canahuati J, Rivera LL, Dewey KG. Effects of age of introduction of complementary foods on infant breast milk intake, total energy intake, and growth: a randomised intervention study in Honduras. *Lancet.* 1994;344:288-293.
24. Birch LL, Deysher M. Conditioned and unconditioned caloric compensation: evidence for self-regulation of food intake in young children. *Learning and Motivation.* 1985;16:341-355.
25. Birch LL, Deysher M. Caloric compensation and sensory specific satiety: evidence for self regulation of food intake by young children. *Appetite.* 1986;7:323-331.
26. Birch LL, Johnson SL, Jones MB, Peters JC. Effects of a nonenergy fat substitute on children's energy and macronutrient intake. *The American Journal of Clinical Nutrition.* 1993;58:326-333.
27. Johnson SL, Birch LL. Parents' and children's adiposity and eating style. *Pediatrics.* 1994;94:653-661.
28. Birch LL, Fisher JO. Mothers' child-feeding practices influence daughters' eating and weight. *The American Journal of Clinical Nutrition.* 2000;71:1054-1061.
29. Wright P. Learning experiences in feeding behaviour during infancy. *Journal of Psychosomatic Research.* 1988;32:613-619.
30. Birch LL, Gunder L, Grimm-Thomas K, Laing DG. Infants' consumption of a new food enhances acceptance of similar foods. *Appetite.* 1998;30:283-295.
31. Sullivan SA, Birch LL. Infant dietary experience and acceptance of solid foods. *Pediatrics.* 1994; 93:271-277.
32. Sullivan SA, Birch LL. Pass the sugar, pass the salt: experience dictates preference. *Developmental Psychology.* 1990;26:546-551.
33. Wardle J, Cooke LJ, Gibson EL, Sapochnik M, Sheiham A, Lawson M. Increasing children's acceptance of vegetables; a randomized trial of parent-led exposure. *Appetite.* 2003;40:155-162.
34. Hearn MD, Baranowski T, Baranowski J, et al. Environmental determinants of behavior among children: availability and accessibility of fruits and vegetables. *Journal of Health Education.* 1998; 29:26-32.

35. Kratt P, Reynolds K, Shewchuk R. The role of availability as a moderator of family fruit and vegetable consumption. *Health Education & Behavior: The Official Publication of the Society for Public Health Education.* 2000;27:471-482.
36. Cullen KW, Baranowski T, Owens E, Marsh T, Rittenberry L, de Moor C. Availability, accessibility, and preferences for fruit, 100% fruit juice, and vegetables influence children's dietary behavior. *Health Education & Behavior: The Official Publication of the Society for Public Health Education.* 2003;30:615-626.
37. Fisher JO, Mitchell DC, Smiciklas-Wright H, Mannino ML, Birch LL. Meeting calcium recommendations during middle childhood reflects mother-daughter beverage choices and predicts bone mineral status. *The American Journal of Clinical Nutrition.* 2004;79:698-706.
38. Rolls BJ, Engell D, Birch LL. Serving portion size influences 5-year-old but not 3-year-old children's food intakes. *Journal of the American Dietetic Association.* 2000;100:232-234.
39. Orlet Fisher J, Rolls BJ, Birch LL. Children's bite size and intake of an entrée are greater with large portions than with age-appropriate or self-selected portions. *The American Journal of Clinical Nutrition.* 2003;77:1164-1170.
40. Nisbett RE. Determinants of food intake in human obesity. *Science.* 1968;159:1254-1255.
41. Shaw J. The Influence of Type of Food and Method of Presentation on Human Eating Behavior [dissertation]. Philadelphia, Pa: University of Pennsylvania; 1973.
42. Edelman B, Engell D, Bronstein P, Hirsch E. Environmental effects on the intake of overweight and normal-weight men. *Appetite.* 1986;7:71-83.
43. Engell D, Kramer M, Zaring D, Birch L, Rolls BJ. Effects of serving size on food intake in children and adults. *Obesity Research.* 1995;3(suppl 3):381S.
44. Diliberti N, Bordi PL, Conklin MT, Roe LS, Rolls BJ. Increased portion size leads to increased energy intake in a restaurant meal. *Obesity Research.* 2004;12:562-568.
45. Rolls BJ, Roe LS, Kral TV, Meengs JS, Wall DE. Increasing the portion size of a packaged snack increases energy intake in men and women. *Appetite.* 2004;42:63-69.
46. Rolls BJ, Morris EL, Roe LS. Portion size of food affects energy intake in normal-weight and overweight men and women. *The American Journal of Clinical Nutrition.* 2002;76:1207-1213.
47. Huang TT, Howarth NC, Lin BH, Roberts SB, McCrory MA. Energy intake and meal portions: associations with BMI percentile in U.S. children. *Obesity Research.* 2004;12:1875-1885.
48. Smiciklas-Wright H, Mitchell DC, Mickle SJ, Goldman JD, Cook A. Foods commonly eaten in the United States, 1989-1991 and 1994-1996: are portion sizes changing? *Journal of the American Dietetic Association.* 2003;103:41-47.
49. Birch LL. Effects of peer models' food choices and eating behaviors on preschoolers' food preferences. *Child Development.* 1980;51:489-496.
50. Hendy HM, Raudenbush B. Effectiveness of teacher modeling to encourage food acceptance in preschool children. *Appetite.* 2000;34:61-76.
51. Hendy HM. Effectiveness of trained peer models to encourage food acceptance in preschool children. *Appetite.* 2002;39:217-225.
52. Lee S, Reicks M. Environmental and behavioral factors are associated with the calcium intake of low-income adolescent girls. *Journal of the American Dietetic Association.* 2003;103:1526-1529.
53. Cullen KW, Baranowski T, Rittenberry L, Cosart C, Hebert D, de Moor C. Child-reported family and peer influences on fruit, juice and vegetable consumption: reliability and validity of measures. *Health Education Research.* 2001;16:187-200.
54. Young EM, Fors SW, Hayes DM. Associations between perceived parent behaviors and middle school student fruit and vegetable consumption. *Journal of Nutrition Education and Behavior.* 2004;36:2-8.
55. Birch LL, Zimmerman SI, Hind H. The influence of social-affective context on the formation of children's food preferences. *Child Development.* 1980;51:856-861.
56. Birch LL, Birch D, Marlin DW, Kramer L. Effects of instrumental consumption on children's food preference. *Appetite.* 1982;3:125-134.
57. Birch LL, Marlin DW, Rotter J. Eating as the "means" activity in a contingency: effects on young children's food preference. *Child Development.* 1984;55:432-439.

58. Fisher JO, Mitchell DC, Smiciklas-Wright H, Birch LL. Parental influences on young girls' fruit and vegetable, micronutrient, and fat intakes. *Journal of the American Dietetic Association.* 2002;102:58-64.
59. Galloway AT, Fiorito L, Lee Y, Birch LL. Parental pressure, dietary patterns, and weight status among girls who are "picky eaters." *Journal of the American Dietetic Association.* 2005;105:541-548.
60. Wardle J, Carnell S, Cooke L. Parental control over feeding and children's fruit and vegetable intake: how are they related? *Journal of the American Dietetic Association.* 2005;105:227-232.
61. Lee Y, Birch LL. Diet quality, nutrient intake, weight status, and feeding environments of girls meeting or exceeding the American Academy of Pediatrics recommendations for total dietary fat. *Minerva Pediatrica.* 2002;54:179-186.
62. Birch LL, McPheee L, Shoba BC, Steinberg L, Krehbiel R. "Clean up your plate": effects of child feeding practices on the conditioning of meal size. *Learning and Motivation.* 1987;18:301-317.
63. Fisher JO, Birch LL. Restricting access to palatable foods affects children's behavioral response, food selection, and intake. *The American Journal of Clinical Nutrition.* 1999;69:1264-1272.
64. Corwin RL, Wojnicki FH, Fisher JO, Dimitriou SG, Rice HB, Young MA. Limited access to a dietary fat option affects ingestive behavior but not body composition in male rats. *Physiology & Behavior.* 1998;65:545-553.
65. Birch LL, Fisher JO, Davison KK. Learning to overeat: maternal use of restrictive feeding practices promotes girls' eating in the absence of hunger. *The American Journal of Clinical Nutrition.* 2003; 78:215-220.
66. Francis LA, Birch LL. Maternal weight status modulates the effects of restriction on daughters' eating and weight. *International Journal of Obesity and Related Metabolic Disorders: Journal of the International Association for the Study of Obesity.* 2005;29:942-949.
67. Faith MS, Berkowitz RI, Stallings VA, Kerns J, Storey M, Stunkard AJ. Parental feeding attitudes and styles and child body mass index: prospective analysis of a gene-environment interaction. *Pediatrics.* 2004;114:e429-e346.
68. Spruijt-Metz D, Lindquist CH, Birch LL, Fisher JO, Goran MI. Relation between mothers' child-feeding practices and children's adiposity. *The American Journal of Clinical Nutrition.* 2002;75:581-586.
69. Robinson TN, Kiernan M, Matheson DM, Haydel KF. Is parental control over children's eating associated with childhood obesity? Results from a population-based sample of third graders. *Obesity Research.* 2001;9:306-312.
70. Wardle J, Sanderson S, Guthrie CA, Rapoport L, Plomin R. Parental feeding style and the inter-generational transmission of obesity risk. *Obesity Research.* 2002;10:453-462.
71. Francis LA, Hofer SM, Birch LL. Predictors of maternal child-feeding style: maternal and child characteristics. *Appetite.* 2001;37:231-243.
72. Baughcum AE, Burklow KA, Deeks CM, Powers SW, Whitaker RC. Maternal feeding practices and childhood obesity: a focus group study of low-income mothers. *Archives of Pediatrics & Adolescent Medicine.* 1998;152:1010-1014.
73. Bentley M, Gavin L, Black MM, Teti L. Infant feeding practices of low-income, African-American, adolescent mothers: an ecological, multigenerational perspective. *Social Science & Medicine (1982).* 1999;49:1085-1100.
74. Bronner YL, Gross SM, Caulfield L, et al. Early introduction of solid foods among urban African-American participants in WIC. *Journal of the American Dietetic Association.* 1999;99:457-461.
75. Barton SJ. Infant feeding practices of low-income rural mothers. *MCN. The American Journal of Maternal Child Nursing.* 2001;26:93-97.
76. Maynard LM, Galuska DA, Blanck HM, Serdula MK. Maternal perceptions of weight status of children. *Pediatrics.* 2003;111(5, pt 2):1226-1231.
77. Baughcum AE, Chamberlin LA, Deeks CM, Powers SW, Whitaker RC. Maternal perceptions of overweight preschool children. *Pediatrics.* 2000;106:1380-1386.
78. Anderson CB, Hughes SO, Fisher JO, Nicklas TA. Cross-cultural equivalence of feeding beliefs and practices: the psychometric properties of the child feeding questionnaire among blacks and Hispanics. *Preventive Medicine.* 2005;41:521-531.

79. Fisher JO, Patrick H, Butte NF. *Restrictive Child Feeding Practices Are Associated With Children's Eating Behavior and Evaluation in Hispanic Families.* Atlanta, Ga: Society for Research in Child Development; 2005.
80. Musher-Eizenman D, Holub SC. *Parenting Styles, Feeding Practices, and Child Eating Outcomes: A Mediational Model.* Atlanta, Ga: Society for Research in Child Development; 2005.
81. Johnson SL. Improving preschoolers' self-regulation of energy intake. *Pediatrics.* 2000;106:1429-1435.
82. Hughes SO, Power TG, Orlet Fisher J, Mueller S, Nicklas TA. Revisiting a neglected construct: parenting styles in a child-feeding context. *Appetite.* 2005;44:83-92.

Do Race and Ethnicity Influence Parents' Feeding Strategies, Perceptions of and Concerns About Child Weight, and Intervention Techniques?

Bettylou Sherry, PhD, RD
Kelley S. Scanlon, PhD, RD
Elizabeth Barden, PhD
Jan Kallio, MS, RD, LDN

Introduction

The prevalence of overweight among adolescents and children in the United States has substantially increased over the past 2 decades.[1] Among preschool-age children, the prevalence of overweight (sex-specific body mass index-for-age $\geq$ 95th percentile) increased from 7.2% to 10.3% between the periods 1976-1980 and 1999-2002.[1,2] This increase in overweight among children was accompanied by increases in health risks and comorbidities experienced during childhood and/or adulthood.[3-12]

As the prevalence of pediatric overweight continues to increase in the United States and other developed countries, healthcare professionals are challenged to address this important public health problem. We must develop interventions that are evidence-based and culturally appropriate. In addition, we need to identify the most effective ways to implement these interventions.[13]

Parents play an important role in the development of their children's eating behaviors, food preferences and energy intake.[14] For example, parents commonly restrict their children's access to sweets, snack foods and other foods they believe are unhealthy, and encourage or even pressure them to eat healthy foods.[15] A growing body of evidence suggests that these well-intended parental child-feeding strategies — restriction in particular — may actually contribute to overeating and the development of pediatric overweight.[16]

Studies of predominantly white, middle-income families showed that parents who control their children's intake of high-fat, energy-dense foods may actually spur the development of their children's preferences for these foods, limit their acceptance of a variety of foods, and disrupt their natural ability to self-regulate energy intake by altering their responsiveness to internal hunger and satiety cues.[17-20] A 2-year follow-up study of 5-year-old white girls demonstrated that parental restriction of intake was positively associated with a high intake of snack foods in the absence of hunger at 7 years of age. This study also found that eating in the absence of hunger at 5 years of age and 7 years of age was associated with overweight at those respective ages.[21] In contrast, a large multiethnic population-based study did not find a significant correlation between parental restriction of foods and body mass index (BMI) in boys or girls.[22]

Associations between parental encouragement during feeding and child energy intake and/or weight are less clear.[23,24] Faith and colleagues[16] conducted a comprehensive review of parental control of child feeding and its associations with child energy intake and child weight status. Among the cross-sectional studies examining the impact of encouragement or pressure to eat, they found 6 studies reported a positive correlation, yet 6 other studies found either no correlation or a negative correlation with child energy intake or BMI.[16]

One area that has received little attention by researchers is the influence of race and ethnicity on the strategies that parents use to feed their children and parents' perceptions of, and concerns about, their children's weight status. Understanding cultural differences in feeding and weight may facilitate the design of interventions aimed at improving children's diets and reducing the prevalence of obesity. While some effective strategies to reduce child obesity have been identified for a particular racial or ethnic group, these approaches need to be reevaluated before being applied to another racial or ethnic group.

This chapter examines the relevant research to determine if race and/or ethnicity have an influence on the following factors:

- Parental child-feeding goals and practices
- Parents' perceptions of, and concerns about, their children's weight
- Parental and program staff perceptions of motivators of behavioral change techniques used in interventions to improve diet and prevent child obesity

The Literature Review

Methodology

To identify published literature for this review we searched the Medline and PubMed databases using the following 5 search terms: "racial/ethnic," "child feeding," "perceptions of overweight," "maternal" and "parental." We further limited our search to studies of children from birth to 7 years of age. We also included findings from final reports of focus groups that were conducted in public health programs and findings from 1 unpublished survey supported by the Centers for Disease Control and Prevention (CDC). (AL May, M Donohue, KS Scanlon, B Sherry, K Dalenius, P Faulkner and LL Birch, unpublished data, 2005.) We extracted only those findings specific to children 7 years of age or less that included more than 1 racial or ethnic group.

Three of the studies we included in our review were based on focus-group research, which does not provide results that can be generalized to the population at large. Therefore, these results are useful only as a first step in identifying differences among racial or ethnic groups. Thus, studies designed to test hypotheses are needed to verify that the racial and ethnic differences preliminarily identified by this focus-group work are, in fact, accurate. It is important to keep this limitation of focus-group work in mind when reading this chapter.

Findings

We identified 5 published studies, 2 reports and 1 unpublished data analysis that met our criteria. The study designs, ages of the children included in the study, sample sizes and areas of focus for these 8 studies are summarized in Table 1.

Table 1. Multiethnic Studies and Unpublished Reports on Parental Child-feeding Strategies, Perceptions of, and Concerns About, Child Weight Status and Motivators for Behavior Change

Study	Design	Child Age	Sample Size	Areas of Study*
May et al (unpublished report)	Survey of low-income mothers in 4 clinics of the Special Supplemental Nutrition Program for Women, Infants, and Children (WIC) in 1 state: non-Hispanic white (79%); non-Hispanic black (6%); Hispanic (15%)	2-5 yr	967	CFS, PC
Sherry et al[25]	12 focus groups: 9 low income (white, black, Hispanic); 3 middle income (predominantly white)	2-<5 yr	101	CFS, PC, MC
Sublet[26]	8 focus groups: white, black; first- and second-marriage families; income not reported	3-7 yr	~40	CFS, PC, MC
Faith et al[29]	Nationally representative survey (National Longitudinal Survey of Youth Data): analyses included black; Hispanic; non-Hispanic; non-black children	3-6 yr	1790	CFS
Taveras et al[31]	Prospective cohort study using questionnaire, >50% middle income: white (76%); black (11%); Hispanic (6%); Asian (4%); multiracial or other (3%)	1 yr	1160	CFS
Barden and Kallio[33]	24 focus groups, low-income WIC in MA: 7 white non-Latina; 6 African-American; 6 Puerto Rican; 5 Dominican	0.5-5 yr	191	PC, MC
Baughcum et al[34]	Survey, median income $60,000-$69,000: white (81%); black (13%); other (6%)	1.9-5 yr	606	PC
Maynard et al[35]	Nationally representative survey (National Health and Nutrition Examination Survey III): all incomes	2-11 yr	5500	PC

*CFS = child-feeding strategies; PC = perceptions and concerns; MC = motivators for behavior change

Parental Child-Feeding Practices

Focus group findings

The focus-group work by Sherry and colleagues[25] was based on a standardized focus-group discussion guide that included a series of questions adapted from the Child Feeding Questionnaire (CFQ),[15] which examines parental child-feeding strategies related to responsibility for feeding, pressure to eat, restriction of feeding and the use of food as a reward or bribe. (The CFQ was developed by Birch and colleagues through research with white and Hispanic parents.) No differences by racial, ethnic or socioeconomic group were identified in the following key themes that emerged from this work:

- All 12 groups described similar goals of providing good nutrition for their children. Most groups wanted their children to avoid eating too many sweets and processed foods. All groups prepared foods that their children liked, accommodated specific requests, and used bribes and rewards (often sweets) to accomplish their feeding goals.
- Parents in 11 of the 12 groups said that they believed that their children were less than truthful when they said they were full, and these mothers then encouraged them to eat more.

These findings suggest that all of the racial, ethnic and income groups included in the focus groups use strategies that can interfere with the promotion of a healthy weight among their children.

Occasionally, focus group participants from a specific racial or ethnic group raised an issue that was not directly questioned or independently discussed in the other groups — and, therefore, it is unclear if the issue was relevant for the other groups. For example, the focus groups of Hispanic mothers emphasized the importance of cultural foods in the diets of their children, but the topic of foods specific to a culture was not specifically questioned or spontaneously raised in focus groups of non-Hispanic mothers.

In another study that consisted of 8 focus groups conducted in December 2001, Sublet identified very few racial or ethnic differences in parental child-feeding goals and practices.[26] In these focus groups, most parents said that dinner was simultaneously the best and worst time of day. While it was an opportunity for the family to share food and conversation, it was also chaotic and stressful. Parents expressed the opinion that they are responsible for providing a nutritious meal for the family and making sure that the children consume enough food. In their attempts to provide healthy meals, parents said that they felt constrained by time and by the availability of "healthy foods." Parents also indicated that they are unlikely to stop purchasing and serving "unhealthy foods" that the family enjoys eating unless their doctor asked them not to serve those particular foods or the products were actually pulled from the market.

According to Sublet,[26] it appeared that the parents who participated in the focus groups were not aware of the public health crisis of pediatric obesity in the United States and did not seem to understand the potential negative consequences of childhood obesity. Several of the parents in the focus groups were overweight themselves. Based on the statements made during the focus groups, first-time parents appeared to be concerned about providing nutritious food to their children; however, the parents who also had older children in the home seemed to place less emphasis on providing healthy foods to their younger children.

This study did note a few racial and ethnic differences in child-feeding practices that emerged in the focus groups:

- Black parents reported that they typically included "soul" (not defined) foods in their diets, while white parents did not mention this term
- Black parents reported frying foods more than did white parents
- Black parents expressed more hesitancy about using the child-feeding guide, *Division of Responsibility for Child-feeding Principle,* promoted by Satter[27] and Dietz and Stern,[28] than did white parents. Black parents said that they did not feel their child was mature enough to decide how much to eat and when to eat. Although white parents also expressed a similar concern, several of them indicated that they believed their children could decide how much food to eat.

Quantitative findings

To examine differences among mothers in the freedom they allow their children to select the foods they consume, Faith and colleagues[29] used data from the National Longitudinal Survey of Youth (NLSY), which includes an overrepresentation of children born to mothers who are relatively young, less educated, disadvantaged and members of minority groups. These researchers found that non-black/non-Hispanic mothers allowed their children to make more choices about the food they ate at breakfast and lunch than did the black or Hispanic mothers (mean 3.2 ± 0.03 SD for non-black/non-Hispanic mothers vs mean 2.0 ± 0.05 and mean 2.9 ± 0.04 for black and Hispanic mothers, respectively; $P<0.001$). The amount of choice that mothers allowed their children in selecting the foods they consumed was quantified categorically as follows: 1 = no choice; 2 = little choice; 3 = some choice and 4 = a great deal of choice.

In another study, May and colleagues (AL May, M Donohue, KS Scanlon, B Sherry, K Dalenius, P Faulkner and LL Birch, unpublished data, 2005) examined child-feeding strategies of mothers participating in the Special Supplemental Nutrition Program for Women, Infants and Children (WIC) program to examine their child-feeding strategies. The survey questions were adapted from the CFQ.[15] More than 90% of the mothers surveyed — regardless of their race or ethnic group — reported that they restricted their preschool-age child from eating too many sweets, junk foods or favorite foods, and pressured their young child to eat enough food and sufficient amounts of the right types of foods. More than 90% of black and Hispanic mothers, compared to 76% of white mothers, reported that they pressured their child to eat all the food on his or her plate.

Nationally representative data from the 2004 National Immunization Survey[30] show that the rate of breastfeeding varies by race and ethnicity. It is lower for black children (55%) than it is for white (74%), Hispanic (78%), Native American (69%), Asian (79%) and Native Hawaiian or Pacific Islander (81%) children. Based on the results of other studies, the breastfeeding behavior of the mother appears to have an important influence on child-feeding practices:

- A study by Taveras and colleagues[31] found that the longer the mother breastfed her infant, the less likely she was to restrict the child's intake of food at 1 year of age. This association remained even after adjusting for demographic, social, economic and anthropometric predictors of breastfeeding, including the mother's race and ethnic group.
- A study of low-income, non-Hispanic white, non-Hispanic black and Hispanic children identified racial and ethnic differences in the protective dose-response relationship between the duration of breastfeeding and the risk of overweight. A significant protective effect was only found among the non-Hispanic white children.[32]

Summary of results on parent child-feeding practices

In summary, the focus-group studies we reviewed suggest that there are similarities among parents in their desire to provide good nutrition for their children that cross racial, ethnic and income groups. Furthermore, mothers from all racial and ethnic groups reported that they use bribes and rewards and prepare foods that their children request to accomplish their feeding goals. Our review revealed differences in the foods consumed among racial and ethnic groups due to the inclusion of culturally specific foods in some groups' diets. Results from surveys and focus groups suggest that white parents give their children more responsibility for mealtime food choices and are less likely to pressure their children to eat than are black and Hispanic parents. Black mothers are less likely to breastfeed their infants than are white, Hispanic, Native American or Asian mothers. This difference in breastfeeding practices, therefore, may affect ethnic differences in parental control of child feeding since breastfeeding may be associated with less parental control of child feeding at a later age. Other differences in racial- or ethnic-group specific child-feeding behaviors still need to be clarified.

Parental Perceptions and Concerns About Child Weight Status

Focus group results

The results of the focus-group work of Sherry and colleagues[25] showed that all of the groups of low-income mothers were concerned about the possibility of their child being underweight. In addition, all of the groups of white mothers and one group of black mothers cited overweight as another concern. Hispanic mothers believed that the good health of their children and the kinds of foods that their children ate were more important than their weight, but they, too, did not want their children to be either underweight or overweight. Middle-income white mothers expressed concerns about their children developing eating disorders and said that they wanted to instill good eating habits in their children early in life. Black mothers generally believed that their children would eventually outgrow any weight problem, and that weighing more in childhood was actually healthy.

This focus-group study identified several potential racial and ethnic differences regarding the role of heredity versus the role of environment in the development of overweight:

- Seven of the 12 groups (3 low-income and 3 middle-income white groups and 1 low-income black group) said that they thought that a combination of genetics and environmental factors determines a child's weight
- Two groups of low-income black mothers cited genetics as the key determinant of a child's weight
- Two low-income Hispanic groups reported that the environment is the key determinant of a child's weight. The third low-income Hispanic group did not respond to this question.

In addition to the responses that Sherry and colleagues obtained from participants during the focus groups, they asked the mothers to define overweight by viewing a series of 7 sequentially numbered schematic drawings of boys and girls, which ranged from very thin (drawing 1) to very overweight (drawing 7), with the middle child (drawing 4) depicting the "ideal" weight status. Mothers were asked to select the drawing that best met their definition of overweight. The drawing most frequently selected by the mothers was 6 (Table 2). One third of the mothers in each of the low-income white and Hispanic groups (32% and 33%, respectively) selected drawing 5 as the overweight child. In contrast, one fifth of the black (21%) and the middle-income white (18%) mothers selected drawing 7 as representative of an overweight child. Both the low-income black mothers and the middle-income white mothers selected drawings 6 and 7 as representative of an overweight child more frequently (96% and 83%, respectively) than did the low-income white (68%) and Hispanic (63%) mothers.

Table 2. Percentage of Mothers Selecting Specific Drawings of Children as Representative of "Overweight"[25]

Mothers were shown the following schematic drawings* ranging from very thin (#1) to very overweight (#7), with the child #4 depicting "ideal" weight status

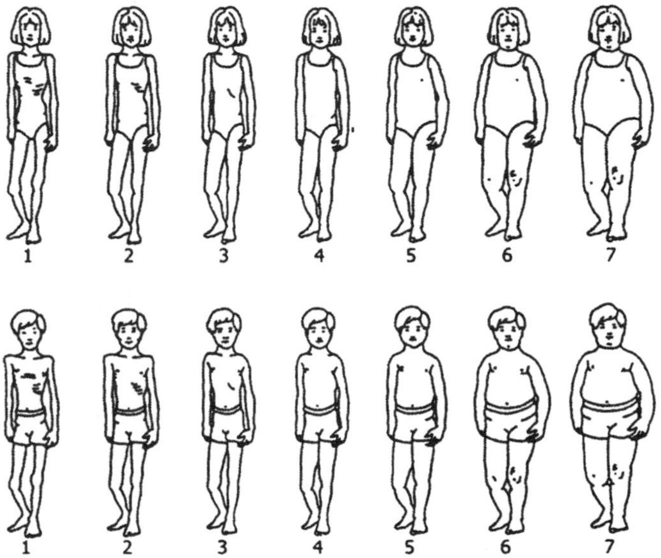

Racial/Ethnic and Income Category	Sample Size	Percentage of Mothers Selecting Drawings as Cut Point for Overweight		
		Child #5	Child #6	Child #7
Low-income Caucasian	22	32	59	9
Low-income African American	24	4	75	21
Low-income Hispanic American	27	33	59	7
Middle-income Caucasian	28	15	67	18

*Source: Collins ME. Body figure perceptions and preferences among pre-adolescent children. *International Journal of Eating Disorders.* 1991;10:199-208. Copyright © 1991, by John Wiley & Sons, Inc. Reprinted with permission.

In contrast, Barden and Kallio[33] reported that there were few racial and ethnic differences in perceptions of overweight among the white non-Latina, black, Puerto Rican and Dominican mothers in their focus groups. The study results showed the following:

- Most of the participating mothers believed that it is possible for children less than 5 years of age to be overweight
- For the most part, the mothers were familiar with the health risks associated with a child being overweight
- Most mothers reported that they did not believe that their own children were overweight, and they would rely on a health professional to diagnose this

The mothers commented that they received conflicting information from their pediatricians and WIC professionals/nutrition counselors about whether their child was overweight, and therefore they believed these professionals used different charts to assess their child's weight. When mothers perceived that information was in conflict, they said that they "believed what they wanted to believe." In general, mothers from all 4 racial and ethnic groups seemed to want to believe that their child was not overweight because they feel it is a very difficult problem to resolve. Furthermore, Barden and Kallio found that all participating mothers perceived that being overweight is determined primarily by heredity, and that presented a key barrier to intervention with an overweight child.

Quantitative analyses findings

In the study conducted by May and colleagues (AL May, M Donohue, KS Scanlon, B Sherry, K Dalenius, P Faulkner and LL Birch, unpublished data, 2005), some 29% of low-income white mothers, compared to 42% of low-income black and 53% of low-income Hispanic mothers, reported that they were concerned about their child becoming overweight. Mothers of children who were already overweight were about 3 times more likely to express concern about child overweight than were mothers of children who were not overweight. Furthermore, when adjusted for race and ethnicity, maternal concern for overweight was positively associated with maternal restriction of specific foods. The researchers also asked mothers to classify the weight status of their child, and only about 21% of mothers correctly classified their child as overweight based on direct weight-for-height measurement. An equal percentage of white and Hispanic mothers (23%) classified their overweight children correctly. None of the 6 overweight black children were classified as overweight by his or her mother, but the sample of black children was small (n = 53) compared to the Hispanic (n = 143) and white (n = 756) samples (AL May, M Donohue, KS Scanlon, B Sherry, K Dalenius, P Faulkner and LL Birch, unpublished data, 2005).

In the study conducted by Baughcum and colleagues,[34] about 20% of the 99 mothers surveyed who had overweight children correctly perceived their child as being overweight, although 95% of obese mothers correctly defined themselves as overweight. Among the mothers with overweight children, the researchers found an association between a low level of maternal education and mothers' incorrect perceptions of their child's weight status, after controlling for family income, maternal obesity, maternal age, maternal smoking, child's age, child's race and gender of the child.

In contrast, using data from the third National Health and Nutrition Examination Survey, Maynard and colleagues[35] found that 67% of mothers correctly classified their overweight children as overweight using standardized growth charts.[36] The researchers measured the height and weight of a nationally representative sample of children 2 to 11 years of age and subsequently compared the children's weight status to their mothers' perceptions of their weight. Neither race nor ethnicity was a significant predictor of the mother's misclassification of her overweight child as "about the right weight" or "underweight," or of her misclassification of her at-risk-for-overweight child as already "overweight."[35]

Summary of results on parental perceptions of and concerns about weight status

In summary, misclassification of their children's weight by their mothers appears to vary widely. Focus-group work based only on mothers' responses to a series of schematic drawings of children ranging from underweight to overweight suggests that the weight at which mothers consider a child to be overweight actually is higher than overweight as defined by standardized growth charts. More middle-income white and low-income black mothers defined drawings 6 and 7 as overweight than did low-income white and low-income Hispanic mothers. In contrast, the latter 2 groups were more likely to choose drawing 5 as representative of an overweight child.[25]

However, the results from one survey (AL May, M Donohue, KS Scanlon, B Sherry, K Dalenius, P Faulkner and LL Birch, unpublished data, 2005) suggest that low-income black and Hispanic mothers are more concerned than are low-income white mothers about their child becoming overweight. Additionally, maternal concerns about child overweight, independent of race and ethnicity, were determined to be positively associated with mothers' restrictions on the types of food their children eat. Findings regarding mothers' beliefs about the role that heredity plays in the development of overweight in children varied in the focus-group studies: One study found that all racial and ethnic groups perceived heredity as the controlling factor,[33] whereas another study found racial and ethnic group inconsistencies in their perceptions of the role of heredity versus the environment as the controlling factors for overweight.[25] Clearly, this area needs further investigation.

Intervention Techniques: Motivators for Behavior Change

Focus group findings

Three of the focus-group studies discussed in the previous sections (Sherry,[25] Barden and Kallio,[33] and Sublet[26]) reported on motivators for change that provide useful information for developing messages for intervention programs for overweight children. Focus-group work by Sherry and colleagues[25] did not examine motivators for change per se, but several mothers (from all participating racial, ethnic and socioeconomic groups) requested guidance on strategies for persuading their children to eat healthy foods and for balancing the desire for convenience, serving a variety of food and reasonable food costs. The nature of these requests may provide some insight into potential motivators that could encourage mothers to change their child-feeding practices. As a group, the mothers were also interested in obtaining information about age-appropriate portion sizes and who (eg, mother or child?) should determine the appropriate portion size for their children.

Low-income white, black and Hispanic mothers who participated in the focus groups conducted by Barden and Kallio[33] cited many practical obstacles to following the advice given to them on how to resolve the problem of a child being overweight. These obstacles included:

- The lack of time to prepare nutritious foods
- The need to rely on other family members/daycare providers who may not adhere to mothers' restrictions of specific foods

- The cost of healthy foods
- The resistance of family members to eat nutritious foods
- Limited motivation on the part of mothers to exercise and engage their children in physical activity

The mothers said that they would like to receive advice that is realistic and practical so that they could incorporate it into their own lives, given the limits on their finances, time and energy.

Mothers from all racial and ethnic groups offered several suggestions:

- Mothers need to be shown evidence on the growth charts that their child actually is overweight
- Healthcare professionals should initiate discussions on overweight by focusing on positive statements that validate the mother's role. Mothers feel judged when they are approached about their child being overweight and are more likely to listen to messages that they perceive as warm and caring.
- WIC staff should make it clear to mothers that they are working in partnership with them to resolve their child's weight problem. They should use open-ended questions to encourage a dialogue with mothers, especially mothers who are defensive.
- WIC staff (and other healthcare professionals) and pediatricians need to collaborate more on how and when to communicate with parents about a child who is overweight. They then can avoid giving parents conflicting information (for example, when a WIC professional tells a mother that her child is overweight, but the pediatrician tells her that it is "nothing to worry about").
- Information that mothers would find helpful includes guidance on the types of food they should prepare, individual recipes, details on appropriate portion sizes; ideas on how to get "fussy eaters to eat healthy foods"; and suggestions for appropriate exercise goals. The mothers said they would like to receive coupons for fruits and vegetables. A few mothers requested advice on the number of times that they should feed their child each day.

In the focus groups they conducted, Barden and Kallio[33] identified the following preferences by race and ethnicity based on the mothers' responses regarding intervention guidance and advice:

- **White mothers** preferred information based on facts, such as those provided in the growth charts. They liked "direct" and "to-the-point" information and indicated that they wanted to be asked about their opinions on their child's weight. They perceived child overweight as a private issue — preferring to discuss it in individual counseling sessions — and viewed pamphlets as "appealing and helpful" reminders of the advice they had been given.
- **Black mothers** said that they felt that the methods used to assess whether a child is overweight and the nutritional guidance they were given were not appropriate for their ethnicity. The focus group researchers suggested that these mothers may believe that African Americans have a different body type and that their children need more food than do children of other races. As a result, the authors concluded, these mothers may be less likely to adhere to advice from healthcare professionals than from other family members. The black mothers were more likely to perceive a diagnosis from a healthcare professional that their child is overweight as a negative judgment of their skill as a parent than were mothers of other races/ethnicities. Based on the responses of these mothers and the variations in their sociodemographic backgrounds, the authors suggested that black mothers who are less informed about health education may be more receptive to advice if it is given by black WIC staff (or healthcare professionals). Black mothers also reported that they felt educational pamphlets were helpful as reminders of the information and advice they were given by WIC staff, including nutrition counselors, or by other healthcare professionals.
- **Puerto Rican** mothers said that the nutritional advice they are given by healthcare professionals is often inconsistent with the diet of their culture. These mothers reported that the staples of their diet were rice, beans, and meat — and did not include many of the recommended vegetables. These mothers consistently expressed the opinion that being overweight as a young child is healthy. (The study authors felt this might be an historical carryover of high levels of poverty and scarcity of foods; thus, a "well-fed" child may appear to be healthier and better nourished.) In addition, the mothers reported that they prefer to learn about how to resolve the problem of an overweight child through parenting groups rather than individual counseling sessions.

- **Dominican mothers** reported that the nutritional advice they are given often is inconsistent with their cultural diets. Many of these mothers, especially those who were not well acculturated to the United States, perceived an overweight infant as a healthy infant. Like the Puerto Rican mothers, the Dominican mothers preferred to learn about how to manage an overweight child through parenting groups rather than through individual counseling. Barden and Kallio[33] concluded that it may be difficult to determine if these mothers understand and agree to the counseling information and guidance they receive because they seemed reluctant to voice any negative comments within the focus groups.

Barden and Kallio further suggested that their research highlights the importance of structuring discussions with mothers about their child's weight using the following guidelines:

- Express care and concern for the child
- Validate the mother as a good parent
- Acknowledge their child as an individual
- Structure the content so that it is culturally appropriate and based on factual evidence
- Make sure that the messages that come from the healthcare provider and the WIC nutrition counselor are consistent

They conclude that most mothers perceive that helping an overweight child to lose weight and eat healthy foods is an extremely difficult task. The barriers to the resolution of a child's weight problem include feelings of hopelessness and denial, lack of money and time to prepare healthy foods and meals, and lack of control over the child's diet.

Sublet's focus-group work[26] with black and white parents of varying socioeconomic backgrounds identified 2 racial/ethnic differences in motivators for change: The desire for blacks to include cultural foods in the child's diet and the hesitation among blacks to use the *Division of Responsibility for Childfeeding Principle*[27,28] as discussed previously in this chapter. Parents in these focus groups suggested that educational materials should provide specific guidance on issues that would catch parents' attention, such as television viewing by children more than a certain amount of time per day is positively associated with overweight. Parents also said that they would like to have access to recipes, tips for healthy snacks, information about age-appropriate portion sizes and sample menus. The parents who participated in the focus groups reported that when they did not plan meals, they often resorted to serving fast food to their families; thus they considered information on pre-planned meals helpful. These parents also emphasized the importance of not buying the foods that they did not want their children to eat. Sublet[26] recommended that healthcare professionals and other professionals who work with children and their families provide more education about the consequences of childhood obesity to parents to motivate them to change their child-feeding practices.

Summary of results on motivators for behavior change

In summary, key motivators for change for all racial and ethnic groups include practical strategies that help mothers balance food convenience and costs while providing a variety of healthy foods that their family members like. Mothers from all racial and ethnic groups were interested in obtaining guidance on age-appropriate portion sizes for their children and information on who should assume the responsibility for determining the appropriate portion size for a child. One focus-group study, by Barden and Kallio,[33] reported possible racial and ethnic differences in perceptions and concerns about overweight: Black, Puerto Rican and Dominican mothers may perceive a heavier-weight child as a healthy child. Additionally, these researchers felt that blacks may believe that their children may need more food than other racial groups, that they have a different body type and that the growth charts used by healthcare professionals to evaluate their child are therefore not relevant to their race or ethnicity. Among the specific racial and ethnic differences in beliefs about and preferences for approaches to counseling identified by Barden and Kallio[33]:

- Low-income white mothers preferred factual information and individual counseling sessions, and found educational pamphlets beneficial.
- Low-income black, Puerto Rican and Dominican mothers felt that the nutritional advice they received could have been enhanced by inclusion of culturally preferred foods. The Puerto Rican and Dominican mothers believed that it is healthy for young children to be overweight, and they preferred to receive counseling in group settings.

Discussion

In our research, we identified 8 studies that examined racial and ethnic influences on parents' feeding practices, parental perceptions and concerns about child weight status, and effective interventions to motivate change to prevent overweight. The literature we reviewed suggested that there are few racial and ethnic differences in these 3 areas. However, only 1 of the studies included a nationally representative sample, and that study focused on parental accuracy in classifying the child's weight status.[35] More research is needed to clarify whether the findings in the studies reported here can be generalized to the overall population of parents of young children in the United States.

With regard to parental child-feeding practices, 2 studies[25,26] reported that mothers from all racial and ethnic groups expressed that they:

- Wanted to provide good nutrition for their children
- Used bribes and rewards to attain their feeding goals
- Were challenged when their children would not eat the foods they served
- Wanted to include foods specific to their culture in the diets of their children

A few potentially important racial and ethnic differences were identified related to the freedom that parents allow their young children to choose foods (white and Hispanic parents more than black parents)[29] and the pressure parents place on children to eat all the food on their plates (Hispanic and black parents more than white parents) (AL May, M Donohue, KS Scanlon, B Sherry, K Dalenius, P Faulkner and LL Birch, unpublished data, 2005). We did not find any studies of multiethnic populations that examined parental restrictions on food intake. Studies in this area are needed, given the consistent positive correlation between restriction of child food intake and child weight.[16] Finally, the evidence suggests that breastfeeding reduces parental control of child feeding at later ages[31] and that black mothers are less likely to breastfeed their infants than are mothers from other racial and ethnic groups.[30]

Several themes emerged from our review of these 8 studies regarding race and ethnicity as it relates to parents' perceptions of a child's weight status, parental feeding and intervention possibilities:

- *Variations in maternal misclassification of child weight status.* A study based on nationally representative data collected from 1988-1994 found that 67% of the mothers of overweight children were able to correctly classify their child as overweight, and race and ethnicity were not significant predictors of misclassification.[35] However, 2 other smaller studies found very different levels of misclassification: The study based on data collected in 1998-1999 from a multiethnic, socioeconomically diverse group of mothers found that only 20% of mothers with overweight children correctly classified their child as being overweight[34] and a study from about the same time period by May and colleagues, which used data collected from low-income mothers, found that only 21% of mothers of overweight children correctly classified their child as overweight (AL May, M Donohue, KS Scanlon, B Sherry, K Dalenius, P Faulkner and LL Birch, unpublished data, 2005). These latter 2 studies are based on data collected about 10 years later than the national data used by Maynard and colleagues[35]; however, it is not clear if the differences in misclassification are due to a secular trend or the result of differences in sample sizes and sampling protocols.

- *Variations in maternal peceptions and concerns about child overweight.* Barden and Kallio,[33] Sherry et al[25] and May et al (AL May, M Donohue, KS Scanlon, B Sherry, K Dalenius, P Faulkner and LL Birch, unpublished data, 2005) all reported potential differences in mothers' views regarding what is overweight and healthcare professionals' classification of overweight and their use of specific standards to classify overweight. More research is needed to clarify whether there are racial and ethnic differences. Additionally, Barden and Kallio[33] reported potential racial and ethnic differences in what is a healthy weight, preferred terms for describing overweight and concern about children becoming overweight. Again, further research is needed to clarify these differences.

- *Mothers' perceptions that they receive conflicting information.* Barden and Kallio[33] heard comments from mothers that they believe the information about their child's weight status that they receive from public health program staff (eg, WIC) is different than what they receive from their pediatricians.

- *Heredity or environment?* Preliminary data from 1 focus-group study[25] suggest that low-income black mothers believe that genetics is a more important factor than the environment as a weight-determining factor; Hispanic mothers consider the environment to be the key determinant.

In contrast, Barden and Kallio[33] found that low-income Hispanic, black and white mothers all believed that a child's weight, including being overweight, is determined primarily by heredity. Further investigation is needed to understand variations among racial and ethnic groups in parents' perceptions of the roles that genetics and the environment play in the development of overweight.

- *Mothers want guidance to help them feed their families.* Mothers in all racial and ethnic groups included in this review reported that they need practical advice to help them find a balance among convenience, providing a variety of healthy foods and food costs in feeding their families. Sublet[26] suggested that educational materials for parents should include information about the health risks of obesity for their children. On the other hand, in their work, Barden and Kallio[33] found that mothers already had a relatively clear understanding of the major consequences of obesity in childhood. Across the 8 studies, mothers from all racial and ethnic groups reported that they need guidance on serving age-appropriate portion sizes to their children and a clearer understanding of who should determine their child's portion size.

Barden and Kallio[33] found that culturally appropriate, caring messages are the most effective way to reach *all* mothers. They did find a distinction, however, by racial/ethnic group regarding the most desired methods for counseling: White mothers expressed a preference for individual counseling; black mothers, who are less informed about health issues, may prefer to be counseled by a black professional; and both Puerto Rican and Dominican mothers appear to prefer to be counseled in group sessions rather than individual counseling. Based on these findings and suggestions, counselors and other healthcare professionals should be sensitive to the needs and wishes of mothers; involving them in the development of an intervention plan may increase the probability of the success of that intervention.

Summary and Conclusions

Our analysis of the 8 studies we identified through a literature review identified possible racial and ethnic differences in the following areas:

- The freedom that mothers allow their children to choose foods
- Mothers' perceptions of, and concerns about, child overweight
- Mothers' beliefs about what a healthy weight is
- The approaches mothers prefer to engage them to effectively prevent and manage child overweight

All of these potential differences should be examined further using nationally representative samples or through randomized trials. In particular, research that crosses the socioeconomic strata within ethnic groups is needed. Many of the focus-group studies conducted with black and Hispanic families are limited only to a low-income population. More research also is needed to clarify whether there are specific differences within ethnic groups, for example, between Mexican Americans and Puerto Ricans.

The effectiveness of child-feeding interventions needs to be tested and evaluated across racial, ethnic and socioeconomic groups. After the most effective and culturally appropriate strategies are identified, integrating them within child-feeding intervention programs may improve the impact that public health officials and clinicians can have on reducing childhood obesity in the United States.

The findings and conclusions in this chapter are those of the authors and do not necessarily represent the views of the Centers for the Disease Control and Prevention.

References

1. Ogden CL, Flegal KM, Carroll MD, Johnson CL. Prevalence and trends in overweight among US children and adolescents 1999-2000. *Journal of the American Medical Association.* 2002;288:1728-1732.
2. Hedley AA, Ogden CL, Johnson CL, Carroll MD, Curtin LR, Flegal KM. Prevalence of overweight and obesity among US children, adolescents, and adults, 1999-2002. *Journal of the American Medical Association.* 2004;291:2847-2850.
3. Must A. Morbidity and mortality associated with elevated body weight in children and adolescents. *American Journal of Clinical Nutrition.* 1996;63:445S-447S.

4. Gutin B, Basch C, Shea S. Blood pressure, fitness and fatness in 5- and 6-year-old children. *Journal of the American Medical Association.* 1990;264:1123-1127.
5. Shear CL, Freedman DS, Burke GL, Harsha DW, Berenson GS. Body fat patterning and blood pressure in children and young adults — the Bogalusa Heart Study. *Hypertension.* 1987;9:236-244.
6. Rames LK, Clark WR, Connor WE, Reiter MA, Laver RM. Normal blood pressures and the evaluation of sustained blood pressure elevation in childhood: the Muscatine study. *Pediatrics.* 1978; 61:245-251.
7. Deschamps I, Desjeuz JF, Machinot S, Rolland F, Lestradet H. Effects of diet and weight loss on plasma glucose, insulin and free fatty acids in obese children. *Pediatric Research.* 1978;12:757-760.
8. Parra A, Schultz RB, Graystone JE, Check DB. Correlative studies in obese children and adolescents concerning body composition and plasma insulin and growth hormone levels. *Pediatric Research.* 1971;5:606-613.
9. Freedman DS, Dietz WH, Srinivasan SR, Brenson GS. The relation of overweight to cardiovascular risk factors among children and adolescents: the Bogalusa Heart Study. *Pediatrics.* 1999;103:1175-1182.
10. Dietz WJ Jr, Gross WC, Kirkpatrick JA Jr. Blount disease (tibia vara): another skeletal disorder associated with childhood obesity. *Journal of Pediatrics.* 1982;101:735-737.
11. Kelsey JL, Acheson RM, Keggi KJ. The body build of patients with slipped capital femoral epiphysis. *American Journal of Diseases of Children.* 1972;124:276-281.
12. Strauss RS. Childhood obesity and self-esteem. *Pediatrics.* 2000;105(1):e15. Available at: http://pediatrics.aappublications.org/cgi/content/full/105/1/e15. Accessed March 24, 2005.
13. Sherry B. Food behaviors and other strategies to prevent and treat pediatric overweight. *International Journal of Obesity.* 2005;29:S116-S121.
14. Birch LL, Fisher JO. Development of eating behaviors among children and adolescents. *Pediatrics.* 1998;101:539-549.
15. Birch LL, Fisher JO, Grimm-Thomas K, Markey CN, Sawyer R, Johnson SL. Confirmatory factor analysis of child feeding questionnaire: a measure of parental attitudes, beliefs, and practices about child feeding and obesity proneness. *Appetite.* 2001;36:201-210.
16. Faith MS, Scanlon KS, Birch LL, Francis LA, Sherry B. Parent-child feeding strategies and their relationship to child eating and weight status. *Obesity Research.* 2004;12:1711-1722.
17. Johnson SL, Birch LL. Parents' and children's adiposity and eating style. *Pediatrics.* 1994;94:653-661.
18. Fisher JO, Birch LL. Restricting access to palatable foods affects children's behavioral response, food selection, and intake. *American Journal of Clinical Nutrition.* 1999;69:1264-1272.
19. Birch LL, Fisher JO. Mothers' child-feeding practices influence daughters' eating and weight. *American Journal of Clinical Nutrition.* 2000;71:1054-1061.
20. Constanzo PR, Woody EZ. Domain-specific parenting styles and their impact on the child's development of particular deviance: the example of obesity proneness. *Journal of the Society of Clinical Psychology.* 1985;3:425-445.
21. Fisher JO, Birch LL. Eating in the absence of hunger and overweight in girls from 5 to 7 y of age. *American Journal of Clinical Nutrition.* 2002;76:226-231.
22. Robinson TN, Kierman M, Matheson DM, Haydel KF. Is parental control over children's eating associated with childhood obesity? Results from a population-based sample. *Obesity Research.* 2001;9:306-312.
23. Klesges RC, Malott JM, Boschee PF, Weber JM. The effects of parental influences on children's food intake, physical activity, and relative weight. *International Journal of Eating Disorders.* 1986;5:335-346.
24. Koivisto U-K, Fellenius J, Sjödjèn P-O. Relations between parental mealtime practices and children's food intake. *Appetite.* 1994;22:245-258.

25. Sherry B, McDivitt J, Birch LL, et al. Attitudes, practices, and concerns about child feeding and child weight status among socioeconomically diverse white, Hispanic, and African-American mothers. *Journal of the American Dietetic Association.* 2004;104:215-221.

26. Sublet V, Oak Ridge Institute for Science and Education. *Report of Focus Groups: Parenting Skills and Childhood Obesity.* Prepared for the Division of Nutrition and Physical Activity, Centers for Disease Control and Prevention, Atlanta, Ga. April 29, 2002.

27. Satter EM. The feeding relationship. *Journal of the American Dietetic Association.* 1986;86:352-356.

28. Dietz WH, Stern L. *American Academy of Pediatrics Guide to Your Child's Nutrition.* New York, NY: Villard Books; 1999.

29. Faith M, Heshka S, Keller KL, et al. Maternal-child feeding patterns and child body weight. *Archives of Pediatrics and Adolescent Medicine.* 2003;157:926-932.

30. National Immunization Survey Data, 2004. Table 1. Breastfeeding rates by sociodemographic factors. Available at: http://www.cdc.gov/breastfeeding/data/NIS_data/index.htm. Accessed August 25, 2005.

31. Taveras EM, Scanlon KS, Birch L, Rifas-Shiman SL, Rich-Edwards JW, Gillman MW. Association of breastfeeding with maternal control of infant feeding at age 1 year. *Pediatrics.* 2004;114:e577-e583. Available at: www.pediatrics.org/cgi/doi/10.1542/peds.2004-0801. Accessed August 25, 2005.

32. Grummer-Strawn LM, Mei Z. Does breastfeeding protect against pediatric overweight? Analysis of longitudinal data from the Centers for Disease Control and Prevention Pediatric Nutrition Surveillance System. *Pediatrics.* 2004;113:e81-e86. Available at: http://pediatrics.aappublications.org/cgi/reprint/113/2/e81. Accessed November 2, 2005.

33. Barden EM, Kallio J. Cultural perspectives on childhood overweight among Hispanic WIC participants in Massachusetts. U.S. Department of Agriculture FY2001 Special Projects Grant Final Report. Boston, Mass, Massachusetts Department of Public Health, 2005.

34. Baughcum AI, Chamberlin LA, Deeks CM, Powers SW, Whitaker RC. Maternal perceptions of overweight preschool children. *Pediatrics.* 2000;106;1380-1386.

35. Maynard LM, Galuska DA, Blank HM, Serdula MK. Maternal perceptions of weight status of children. *Pediatrics.* 2003;111;1226-1231.

36. Kuczmarski RJ, Ogden CL, Guo SS, et al. 2000 CDC growth charts for the United States: methods and development. *Vital Health Statistics.* 2002;11(246):1-190.

Eating Behaviors of the Young Child
Prenatal and Postnatal Influences on Healthy Eating

Section 3
Delivery Systems

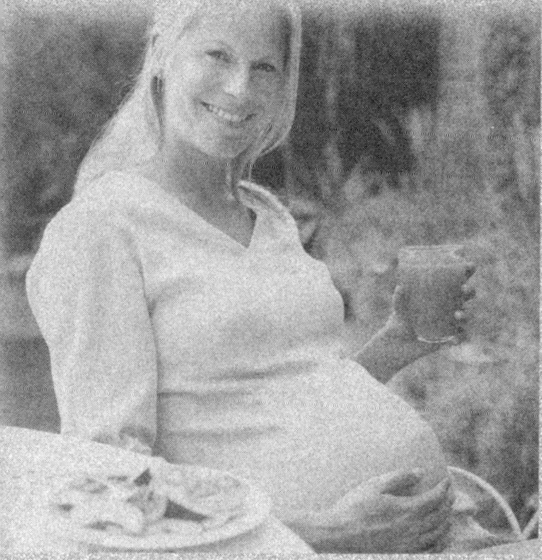

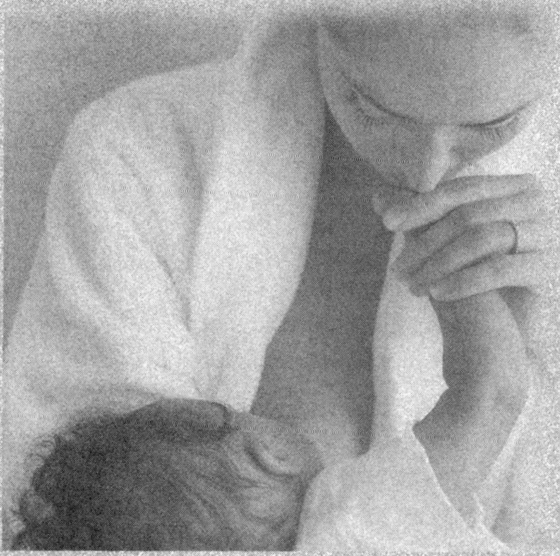

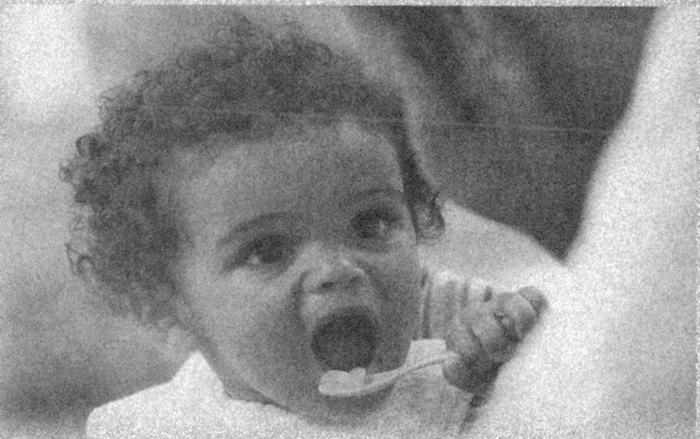

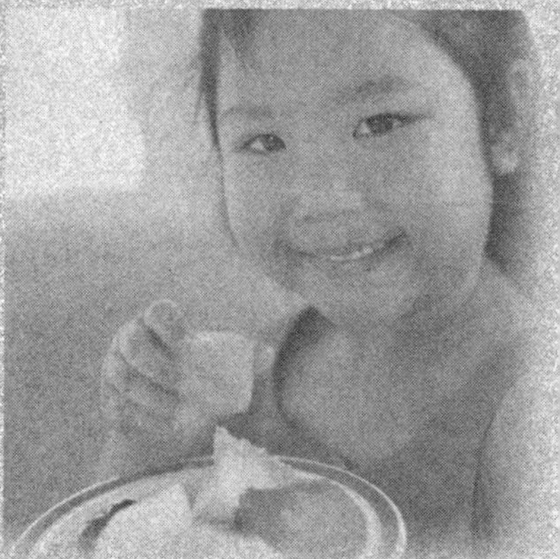

Abstracts From Section 3 Delivery Systems

Supporting Parents Around Feeding and Eating in Early Childhood

Jon Korfmacher, PhD

There is a long history in the United States of providing advice and guidance to parents of young children — in many different forms and from many different experts — to promote healthy child growth and development. In the past 30 years, formal early childhood intervention programs have emerged as one way of providing guidance and support to higher risk families. This paper reviews early childhood interventions in general and presents findings from one intervention trial in particular — the Chicago Doula Project — to illustrate the challenges these programs face in working with parents around issues of feeding and eating.

Motivational Interviewing for Pediatric Obesity: Conceptual Issues and Evidence Review

Ken Resnicow, PhD
Rachel Davis, MPH
Stephen Rollnick, PhD

Counseling by healthcare professionals represents a potentially important intervention for the prevention and treatment of pediatric obesity. One promising approach to weight-control counseling in pediatric practice is motivational interviewing. This article explores conceptual issues related to the application of motivational interviewing for the prevention and treatment of pediatric obesity. Given the paucity of studies on motivational interviewing and pediatric obesity, we examine what is known about the application of motivational interviewing to modify diet, physical activity and other behaviors in children and adolescents. The authors begin with a brief overview of motivational interviewing, describe some nuances of applying this approach to pediatric overweight and conclude with research and clinical recommendations.

Mealtimes and Beyond: Ways of Working With Parents When Eating Difficulties Prevail

Mary Rudolf, MB

By studying young children with failure to thrive — the majority of whom are difficult for parents to feed — it is possible to learn a great deal about eating behavior, how it can go awry, and the resulting difficulties and concerns experienced and expressed by parents. This chapter discusses failure to thrive and how the problem often is handled poorly by healthcare professionals. The author subsequently focuses on the promising work of the Belmont House Growth and Nutrition Team. Established in 1993 in Leeds, England, the Belmont House provides a clinical service to families with babies and young children who are failing to thrive. The chapter discusses the approach and tools employed by the multidisciplinary care team.

Using Childcare Programs as a Portal for Changing the Eating Behaviors of Young Children

Richard Fiene, PhD

In the United States, the majority of preschool-age children spend time each week in childcare settings, and often eat one or more meals there. Childcare programs, therefore, are a natural portal for interventions targeted to young children and their families. This chapter examines findings from a randomized clinical trial on mentoring in childcare and suggests how content relevant to children's eating behaviors could be introduced into the model.

Supporting Parents Around Feeding and Eating in Early Childhood

Jon Korfmacher, PhD

There is a long history in the United States of providing advice and guidance to parents of young children — in many different forms and from many different experts — to promote healthy child growth and development.[1] In the past 30 years, formal early childhood intervention programs have emerged as one way of providing guidance and support to *higher* risk families.[2,3] This paper will briefly review early childhood interventions in general and use findings from one intervention trial in particular — the Chicago Doula Project[4] — to illustrate the challenges these programs face in working with parents around issues of feeding and eating.

What Are Early Childhood Interventions?

"Early childhood intervention" is a label given to prevention and support programs for "at-risk" families that typically begin during the prenatal period or in the first year of a child's life. The family's risk is defined by a number of statistics, including the presence of poverty, first-time parenting or teen parenting.[3] These programs follow many different models and are provided through a number of different venues: home-based (reaching out to the family where they live), center-based (providing childcare and developmental services in a single location or clinic that families travel to), or a mix of the two. The duration of these programs is also variable. Some involve only a few meetings with parents, while others may extend over a period of several years or more.

Early childhood intervention programs often take a "kitchen sink" approach and can intervene with nearly any aspect of a parent's or child's life — from the child's physical health, emotional functioning, cognitive development or school readiness to the parent's mental health and well-being, and the family's economic functioning or social support. They are typically separate from (but may complement) early intervention services for children who have been identified with delays or disabilities, as defined by Part C of the US Federal Individuals with Disabilities Education Improvement Act of 2004. Table 1 summarizes some of the more well-known early childhood intervention programs.[5-9]

Table 1. Early Childhood Intervention Programs

Program Name and Website(s)	Description of Program
Early Head Start[5] (EHS) www.acf.dhhs.gov/programs/hsb/programs/ehs/ehs2.htm ehsnrc.org	An infant and toddler extension of the federally funded preschool Head Start program, EHS was developed in the mid-1990s. Providing center-based or home-based programming (sometimes combining the two), EHS programs follow Head Start performance standards. Some families may enroll prenatally, but most children are enrolled within the first 2 years of life.
Healthy Families America/ Healthy Start[6] www.healthyfamiliesamerica.org	The Healthy Start program model that was initially developed in Hawaii for child abuse prevention was then modified and disseminated under Healthy Families America. Families are enrolled after a child's birth based on a risk screening.
Healthy Steps[7] (Healthy Steps for Young Children) www.healthysteps.org	Developed by the Commonwealth Fund, Healthy Steps uses trained pediatric specialists to provide child development guidance during pediatric care visits. The program is used in different ways depending on local community needs.
Nurse–Family Partnership[8] (NFP) www.nursefamilypartnership.org	Developed and disseminated by David Olds and colleagues, NFP offers home visiting services provided by nurses to first-time mothers from the prenatal period until the child is 2 years of age. NFP has strong empirical support because it was validated across 3 different randomized trials.
Parents as Teachers[9] www.parentsasteachers.org	Parents as Teachers is a home visitation program developed in Missouri in the early 1980s to address school readiness. Parents are supported by home visits, screenings, group meetings and referrals to community services. Families enroll prenatally or in the first year, with services lasting until the child is 3 years of age.

In the United States, early childhood intervention is not a unified system of service delivery, but the programs are a significant part of the landscape of early childhood services — especially for at-risk families. Although there is great diversity to these programs, it is possible to identify some common qualities:

- **Parent as focus.** Most early childhood intervention efforts are targeted at parents. Even center-based programs that provide full-day childcare recognize the significant and central role of the parent in the young child's life. Historically, these programs have focused on the mother as the parent because it often is very difficult to involve fathers.
- **Strengths-based.** Early childhood programs tend to promote healthy development rather than the amelioration of existing concerns or conditions. They work with parents "where they are," assuming that parents are experts on their own children, and that each parent wants what is right for their child. By the very nature of the high-risk populations they target, however, programs tend to enroll noticeable numbers of distressed families with significant social and mental health issues. These families can be very challenging to work with, especially for providers with circumscribed training and resources.
- **Longitudinal.** Early childhood intervention programs often work with families over a period of time (sometimes as long as 5 years) and hope to see long-term impacts from this involvement. Follow-up studies and cost-benefit analyses have demonstrated that these hopes are not misplaced, as long-term benefits have been shown for improved family income, fewer repeat pregnancies, greater school completion levels and fewer behavior problems.[10,11]
- **Flexible.** Even if an early childhood intervention program follows a manual or curriculum, flexibility is highly valued. Two of the most widespread programs, Early Head Start and Healthy Families America, provide general performance standards but dictate very little in the way of specific service content.[5,6] Even manuals that provide session-by-session content can be individualized to meet specific family needs. Ideally, parents and providers decide together the areas on which they will focus. While program staff may see difficulties in areas of child or family well-being where the parent sees none, the *voluntary* nature of these programs dictates that staff respect family beliefs and not pressure guidance on uninterested or unwilling families.

Do These Programs Work?

The research and social service communities have paid considerable attention to the question of whether early childhood intervention programs work. Generally, the answer is yes, but not as well as we would like them to.[3,12] It has become clear that the question is actually too simplistic: it assumes everyone receives uniform treatment and it ignores individual differences in implementation and response to the program. A better question to ask might be: What works, for whom and under what circumstances?[13] This question helps us understand why some families commit to and respond to program services while others drop out of sight soon after enrollment.

One of the crucial tasks for those who design or evaluate intervention services, particularly services for high-risk populations, is to understand why families seek out help. This is particularly important for strengths-based early childhood intervention programs. People rarely enroll in programs because they believe they have a problem that needs to be fixed. Rather, they join because they want some kind of help or support *somehow* with *something.* Often, program designers and staff do not really know what that "something" is; they assume that families will participate enthusiastically because the staff is composed of caring people who offer what seems to be a great opportunity for support. Consider the following exchange with a teenage mother in a comprehensive school-based parent support program[14]:

Interviewer: Why did you decide to join the program?

Mother: They just enrolled me in it. One of my friends was in the program, too. And she talked me into getting into it.

Interviewer: What did you think you could get help with?

Mother: I didn't think I could get help with nothing. I didn't really want help. I really don't ask nobody for help.

Interviewer: So why did you join the program then?

Mother: I don't know 'cause I don't see what they give us…Like I know a program, they give out Pampers and stuff like that. We don't get nothing.

The teen mother did not initially value a psychoeducational intervention, wanting instead more concrete assistance. Contrast the above exchange with the same mother's comments about the program 1 year later:

> *Mother:* [She] ran my case a lot, like "Do right," "Go to class," and now she don't have to tell me to do that because I know that these are things that I want to do for myself... [S]he's praising me, motivating me,...I don't want nobody else to work with me and my child but [her].[14]

In the course of a year, this young mother found meaning in the emotional and motivational support she received from her home visitor. Interviews with the mother and her home visitor provided evidence of the importance of this individualized supportive relationship in the teen's acceptance of the program and the guidance it provided. The formation of a strong and trusting supportive relationship is a crucial element in program success for many early childhood interventions, but this relationship is rarely static. Parents have dynamic responses to early childhood intervention services. That is, their understanding of the program changes over time and service providers must continually monitor and modify their approach to manage these shifts. In other words, there are individual differences in program responses both across participants and for the same participants across time.[14]

Feeding, Eating and Early Childhood Interventions

Feeding and nutrition are important aspects of comprehensive early childhood intervention programs. A baby's weight gain and how well he or she eats are, after all, essential concerns for new parents, and key ways to gauge a baby's health and well-being. In early childhood services, program content typically reflects the child's developmental course. During the early months of a child's life and/or prenatally, programs focus on the benefits of breastfeeding or provide guidance on formula feeding if the mother decides not to exclusively breastfeed. In later months, the focus shifts to the transition to solid foods. As the young child grows and develops more autonomy, the eating habits of a toddler become more prominent, and the programs increasingly focus on the need to provide a varied and healthy diet and establish routines and rituals for mealtimes. Safety issues such as cutting foods to the right size so that they are not a choking hazard also are covered.

Early childhood service providers, however, cover many topics in addition to feeding and eating. A review of popular home visiting curricula, such as the Partners for a Healthy Baby series from Florida State University,[15] or the Nurse–Family Partnership home visitor protocols,[16] shows that only a small percentage of the content is devoted to nutrition, mealtimes, eating, feeding or diet. As noted previously, some families will receive relatively more guidance in this area than others, but only if the provider and the family mutually decide (explicitly or implicitly) that encouraging healthy eating is important and requires attention.

Both families and providers may be reticent to make healthy eating a topic of attention. How a parent feeds a young child is an extremely sensitive topic, for several reasons:

- **Considerable parental self-worth is wrapped up in feeding.** Having a child who eats and looks well-fed is a visible symbol of parenting competence. Parents can feel self-conscious and criticized when they are provided guidance on this issue.
- **Especially with newborns and infants, feeding is an intimate act.** Feeding requires extended periods of close interaction — holding and eye contact — and is a time for mutual exploration by the parent and child.
- **Food choices and the act of eating are vital representations of cultural and familial values.**[17] This is particularly true when the parents are young and still rely heavily on support and advice from their own parents or extended family. Criticizing a parent's feeding style may be seen as criticizing the heritage and history of the family.

In summary, feeding and eating are undeniably important areas of focus in early childhood intervention programs. They are, however, topics that can also invoke discomfort for providers who may be apprehensive about broaching sensitive subjects with parents.[18] Healthcare providers should be mindful of the challenges of dealing with these topics. But being mindful can be difficult when one is also trying to cover many other areas of family and child development in a limited period of time. This is especially true when the healthcare provider does not have specialized training or a well-established curriculum to use as a framework or guide.

Breastfeeding Support by Community-Based Doulas: The Chicago Doula Project

Recent work with the Chicago Doula Project illustrates the complexities of providing feeding and nutrition guidance to young mothers, especially regarding breastfeeding. The Chicago Doula Project employs doulas to work with low-income, young black mothers. Doulas are nonmedical, experienced lay helpers who provide emotional support and comfort to mothers during labor and delivery to improve their birth experience.[19] In the Chicago Doula Project, the doulas were black women from the community who were supervised by a registered nurse. All doulas were mothers themselves who had breastfed their own children and were very committed to promoting breastfeeding and being a positive model to the young women with whom they worked. Each doula received extensive pre-service and in-service training focused on childbirth (and childbirth education), parent support, breastfeeding and child caregiving.

The Chicago Doula Project was built on a model of extended doula support that continues beyond labor and delivery. Doulas work with mothers beginning in the prenatal period to 3 months postpartum to provide guidance in the additional areas of parenting efficacy and child development.[4,20] Although breastfeeding of their infants by the young mothers in the program is an important program objective (and a focus of the program's evaluation), it is only one of many topics doulas cover in their work with the young mothers.

In the Chicago Doula Project, the doulas visited weekly with their clients, either in the home or at the clinic, beginning with the mother's prenatal enrollment until the infant reached 3 months of age. During pregnancy, the doulas taught the young mothers about practices that enhance a fetus' development, such as the importance of nutrition and rest, and attending regular prenatal checkups. Doulas also helped build the mother's self-confidence and support her relationship with the baby growing inside of her. For example, they would encourage mothers to talk to or read to the fetus, and they would engage mothers in activities to show how the fetus responds to sensory input. They assisted mothers with developing a birth plan and discussed with them how to interact with healthcare providers. In addition, the doulas worked with the mothers to plan for the baby's arrival, such as thinking through early child care, living arrangements and newborn needs and, in particular, to prepare for breastfeeding. Whenever possible, the doulas also built relationships with other significant family members, such as the young women's mothers and partners.

During labor and delivery, doulas provided continuous emotional support and physical comfort to the young mothers. They helped them and their families negotiate and understand the healthcare system. After delivery, the doulas facilitated the bonding between mothers and their infants. Doulas encouraged initial breastfeeding, close holding and gentle handling of the newborn.

During the 3 months after birth, the doulas' primary focus was helping the young mothers adjust to life as a parent. For example, doulas:

- Provided support to breastfeeding mothers and encouraged other mothers to follow recommended infant feeding practices.
- Monitored scheduled postpartum and well-baby clinic appointments.
- Encouraged the young mothers to feel good about themselves and take pride in the healthy development of their infants.
- Promoted face-to-face interaction with the infants, suggesting that the mothers listen to their babies' vocalizations, read to them and engage them in back-and-forth "conversations."
- Discussed with mothers their plans for returning to school or work, and encouraged the mothers to set long-term goals for education, employment and family life.

Evaluation of the Chicago Doula Project

The evaluation of the Chicago Doula Project was conducted as a randomized trial.[20] During the second or third trimester of pregnancy, 248 young mothers (21 years of age or younger) were assigned to either a program group that received the services of a doula, or a comparison group that did not. As part of the baseline interview, researchers asked mothers about their background, living situations, and their attitudes and beliefs about parenting. The evaluation tracked program outcomes through follow-up interviews and mother–infant observations conducted immediately after birth, and again when the infants were 4, 12 and 24 months of age. In addition, the evaluation team collected extensive information on program implementation in order to understand how the program was administered across families, including variation in amount of contact, the mother's engagement in the program over time and the topics dicussed during visits. This was done primarily using records kept by the doulas, as well as structured and semi-structured interviews with mothers and doulas about the mothers' experiences in the program and the doulas' views about their roles as helping professionals.

At baseline, program staff asked the young mothers whether they would consider breastfeeding their infant. (The wording of this question was purposefully vague so it would not influence the actual decision-making of mothers.) They also were asked what they perceived to be the advantages and disadvantages of breastfeeding, and whether or not their own mothers breastfed them or any of their siblings.

The majority of mothers assigned to the program group that received doula services (66%) said that they would consider breastfeeding their infant, a number similar to the number of mothers in the comparison group who said they would consider breastfeeding. Although this pronouncement does not necessarily translate into an actual intent to breastfeed, it does suggest that the majority of participating mothers had at least considered the possibility. In addition, almost every mother could report at least one advantage for breastfeeding (Figure 1). More than two thirds of mothers directly linked breastfeeding to the health of the child, often citing specific examples, such as its potential to provide immunity for some illnesses and infections. Nearly 25% of the mothers linked breastfeeding to improvements in brain development and cognitive functioning (Figure 1).

Figure 1. Breastfeeding advantages.

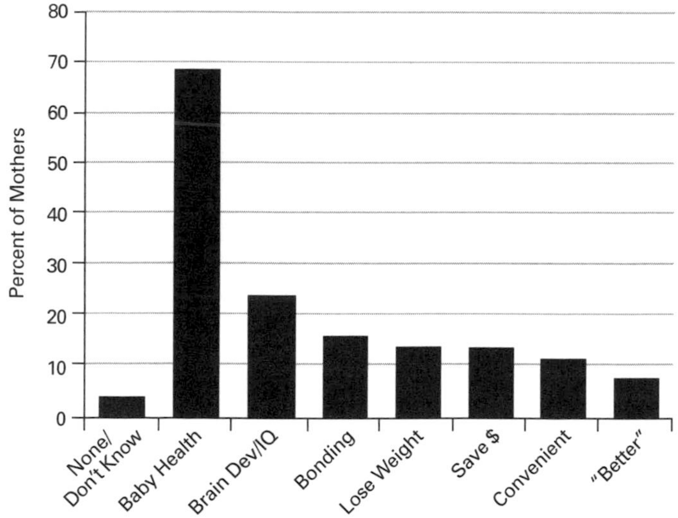

N = 124; some mothers gave >1 response

However, at the same time, 85% of mothers could list at least one disadvantage to breastfeeding (Figure 2). Approximately one third of mothers were worried about pain, and one third had logistical concerns about pumping milk or continuing to breastfeed once they were not home with their child full-time (eg, when they returned to school).

Figure 2. Breastfeeding disadvantages.

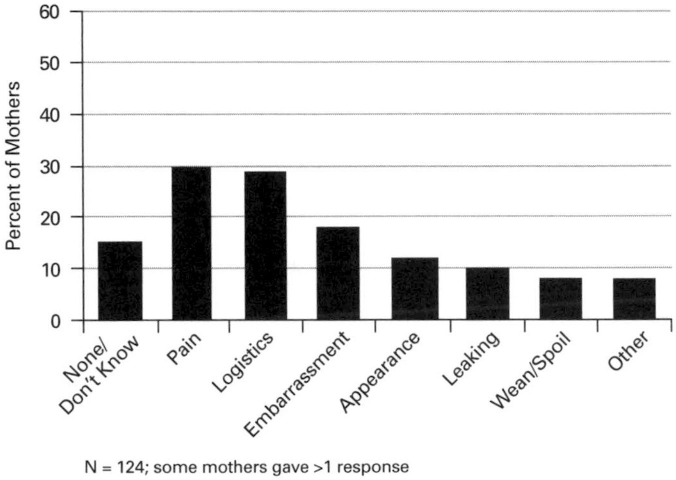

The fact that so many of the mothers could cite at least some benefits associated with breastfeeding suggests that before entering the Chicago Doula Project, the mothers already were receiving some guidance and information about breastfeeding. But the mothers also were very aware of the disadvantages associated with breastfeeding. In other words, these women were fairly ambivalent about breastfeeding, which is not an uncommon attitude among young, black women.[21]

At the follow-up interviews, when babies were 4 months and 12 months of age, the evaluation team asked mothers about the duration and intensity of their breastfeeding. The majority of mothers assigned to the program group that received doula services tried to breastfeed at least once (62%), which was significantly greater than the number of mothers in the comparison group who tried to breastfeed at least once (49%; $P<.05$). However, most of the mothers in both the program group and the comparison group did not continue to breastfeed after an initial attempt, and there was no significant difference between the two groups in the number of mothers who breastfed once they left the hospital (41% vs 34%; Figure 3). Although the mothers in the program group who had the support of a doula breastfed, on average, for a slightly longer period of time than did mothers in the comparison group (5 weeks vs 3 weeks, $P<.05$), by the 4-month follow-up interview, breastfeeding rates (exclusive and nonexclusive) were extremely low for both groups (less than 6%) and almost zero at 12 months. In short, doulas had an effect on the rate of mothers who attempted to breastfeed, but had limited or no effect on the rate of mothers who sustained their breastfeeding once they left the hospital and returned to their daily lives.

Figure 3. Breastfeeding impacts.

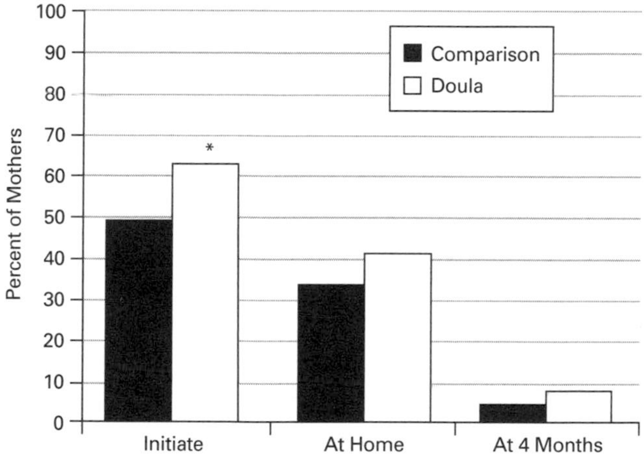

N = 124 in each group
*$P<.05$

The Challenges of Breastfeeding Support

Why was the promotion of sustained breastfeeding so challenging in this program? As part of the study of program implementation, the evaluation team interviewed a subset of participating mothers and their doulas. While the primary focus of the interviews was the nature of the relationship that doulas formed with the mothers, the evaluators also asked the mothers and doulas about what they discussed and did during their time together, with breastfeeding a specific area of questioning. Mothers and doulas were interviewed separately 2 times — once during pregnancy and once after the baby was 2 months of age. Excerpts from these interviews highlight major themes that emerged around how the doulas promoted breastfeeding.

Breastfeeding and Doulas: Themes From the Evaluation Interviews

The first theme to emerge from the interviews was that the doulas were very careful to offer mothers choices and respectfully listen to what they wanted to do, rather than simply pushing them to breastfeed. Consider the comments from this young mother:

> *Young Mother:* She told me well if [formula] is something I wanted to do, to do it, but she would rather totally suggest breastfeed. She told me why, so it wasn't like she just said, "Oh you should just breastfeed," and just left it at that. She explained why I should and I felt it was a good reason. She gave me a choice. It wasn't like she was just pressuring me to do what she wanted me to do.

In the interviews, the mothers frequently mentioned the lack of pressure from doulas to breastfeed as a positive aspect of the program. Although the doulas felt very strongly about the importance of breastfeeding — and saw themselves as advocates for it — they adopted the deliberate strategy of listening to the mothers' desires to show that they understood their circumstances and valued their decision-making processes. Another teen summed it up simply: "She don't talk to me like normal people do. She talks with respect."

The tension between providing information that doulas perceived to be helpful and not wanting to force an issue on the young mothers was played out in many of the interviews. Here, a doula and her client separately discuss the disagreement they had around breastfeeding:

> *Doula:* She said, "I'm not going to do it." I said, "But you haven't even given it a try." She replied, "Why should I try something that I know I'm not going to finish?" And so I tried to go through the whole thing about the baby being healthy. "Well, I had a bottle and I'm pretty healthy. I know other people that had a bottle and they're healthy," she said. So it was just that constant back and forth.

> *Young Mother:* That's the only thing we disagreed about. I didn't do it, I didn't want to go through it...I was just like "hm, hm, hm, hm, hm, hm." I listened to her, and I'm like, "I'm still not doing it." And you know she finally accepted the fact that this girl has made up her mind.

It was clear from the entire interview that this mother felt great fondness towards her doula and she praised her doula in many ways — but she especially appreciated how the doula respected her opinion and refrained from asking her further about something that she had no interest in doing. This respect was crucial to the doula's work with the mother, but it also meant that the doula had to be prepared to let go of issues about which she had strong feelings.

A second theme that emerged from the interviews is that the doulas and the mothers developed close personal relationships with each other, relationships that were different than those typically seen between a young mother and a doctor or nurse. For example, it was not uncommon for both the doulas and the teens to use the word love to describe their emotional bond. Most of the doulas and the mothers reported that they viewed the role of the doula as similar to the role of a family member (such as a big sister, aunt or mother). Serving clients in this capacity, with more permeable professional boundaries, is a hallmark of paraprofessionals and community-based providers in general,[22] but it was likely accentuated for these doulas because of the intimacy of attending the labor and delivery, and the need to be on-call during all hours of the day and night due to labor's unpredictability.

By sharing their own life experiences with the mothers, doulas also helped forge a more personal connection. This was a strategy the doulas used across multiple issues, including breastfeeding. An excerpt from the interviews illustrates this:

> *Young Mother:* Because [my doula] had her baby kind of young...she could understand some of the things I'm going through by me still being a teenager, or whatever, with a baby. So, she was telling me how breastfeeding won't get in the way of my fun and stuff like that. So, she looked at it and back in her time to kind of make it relate closer to mine. So she did help me out.

Doulas used this personal connection to make their advocacy and guidance regarding breastfeeding more real to the young mothers. As a result, the advice they provided on breastfeeding and other infant care issues may have sounded different to the mothers — because it came from someone who felt more like a family member or friend than a doctor or nurse seen only in their own professional setting.

Having this personal role, however, did not necessarily put the doula inside the family. A third theme that emerged from the interviews regarding the challenges of promoting breastfeeding among young mothers is that the doulas had to carefully negotiate the points of view of family members and friends. The following interview excerpt shows this:

> *Doula:* [Her friends] thought it was so gross when we were doing the breastfeeding [video]. "Oh, this is so gross; you're going to do this?" This is what they were saying. She said, "Yeah, it's feeding the baby." And they said, "Oh my God!"

The most influential family member, and the one who was most likely to participate in the doula's visits, was the young mother's own mother (the child's maternal grandmother). Grandmothers often expressed concerns about breastfeeding. Most of the grandmothers did not breastfeed their own children. In fact, only one third of mothers receiving doula services reported that their mother breastfed them and/or their siblings. Many of the grandmothers would be taking care of the child while the young mother worked or returned to school, and they discouraged breastfeeding because of the complications or logistical challenges of feeding the infant when the young mother was not there. The following example shows that the doulas recognized this challenge and worked to get the young mothers to try breastfeeding in the beginning, even it was not sustained:

> *Doula:* That's my main focus now, is to try to push, at least get a feeding in…I think her mom just feels like it's easier, like they all do. You're going back to school; this baby needs a bottle.

When a doula and a maternal grandmother had differences of opinion, the young mother could be caught in the middle of the conflict. Consider this example:

> *Young Mother:* [W]hen she got through telling me how it benefits you and the baby and it's better, I listened to her on that. My mother wanted me to bottle feed. Right now, my mama, we going at it. She's trying to stick the bottle in and I be trying to use myself or whatever. I was really confused, because I wanted to listen to my mother, and then, like I said, by me knowing that it help out the baby and me, I wanted to do that, too. So, that's why I just supplemented, to make my mother happy, and breastfed to make me and my baby happy.

The doula suggested to this young mother that she should not introduce formula when the infant is so young and is breastfeeding, but this guidance had the unfortunate effect of forcing the mother to make a choice. The young mother noted that she listened to the doula's advice, decided she could not do both breastfeeding and bottle feeding, and ultimately chose formula after about 2 months. This example shows how carefully doulas must negotiate these differences of opinion. For the most part, the doulas recognized that the maternal grandmother "trumps" the service provider, and emphasized the importance of respecting the decisions and beliefs of the family, as this example shows:

> *Doula:* If they're there, I try to give to the whole family at the same time. I probably address the matriarch. Whichever it is, grandma or mom, I probably address them even before [the young mother], because I know that they're going to be the real influencing factors whether or not she follows what I say. And to respect it if she doesn't. You know, that's okay, it's a family choice.

In group interviews, the doulas revealed that even though they encouraged the mothers to attempt to breastfeed while in the hospital, they rarely visited the mother at her home immediately after birth to provide any follow-up. As part of the doula training, it was recommended that the doulas visit the mothers at home as soon as possible after birth. Research emphasizes the importance of breastfeeding during the first few days after birth to establish a successful breastfeeding pattern.[23] Collectively, however, the doulas determined that the first week after birth was a time for the young mothers to be with their families. They felt uncomfortable about visiting the home so soon after the birth — it felt intrusive to them.

This is another example of the deliberate trade-offs the doulas made to respect the family's beliefs and feelings. The doulas decided that they could better serve the young mothers overall by taking a step back right after birth, even if it meant missing a valuable window of opportunity to encourage breastfeeding — which was an important desired outcome of the program. It is unclear whether the program could have increased the duration of breastfeeding among participating mothers if the doulas had made earlier postpartum contact. The doulas did not want to put their alliance with the young mother and her family at risk — and the important work to be done in the 3 months following the baby's birth — to test this.

Discussion

As with many early childhood interventions, the Chicago Doula Project uses a model of relationship-based care. A strong, trusting, helping relationship between the doula and the parent provides the building block upon which the mother accepts information and guidance, feels encouraged and supported, views herself as someone who deserves to be valued and respected, and (by extension) sees her infant as deserving of empathy and responsive care.[12] As with many strengths-based programs, the Chicago Doula Project emphasizes that all client families want what is best for the child. The doulas work with the parents to establish mutual goals, rather than tell them what they should do.

Bernstein uses a framework of "mutual competence" to describe the ideal provider–parent relationship in early childhood programs.[24] This framework acknowledges that providers and parents often approach important developmental issues from different vantage points. In a mutual competence model, providers must be willing to accept that families will make decisions that are not in agreement with providers' beliefs and goals, and that these decisions are not based merely on ignorance, resistance or problem behavior. The teen mothers in the Chicago Doula Project, for the most part, understood the benefits of breastfeeding from the outset, but they also were aware of some very real challenges to breastfeeding. Ultimately, they made choices that they felt best fit their family and living situation. If their world did not support exclusive, continued breastfeeding because of peer pressure, family preference and/or an intolerant work or school environment, simply understanding the advantages and mechanics of breastfeeding was not enough to persuade them.

The choices that parents make are always meaningful and adaptive in their own way. This is true of almost any parent feeding behavior. What a provider views as unhealthy or inappropriate (such as a mother who does not follow the child's lead in determining satiety), the parent may see as providing nourishment to the child in the manner that makes the most sense, based on their family context and other factors. The job of providers is to understand the parent's perspective and context — and accept the parent's choices, even if they do not agree with them. It is precisely through this acceptance that the parent feels respected, a sense of trust can grow and a common ground can be found. When parents feel respected and accepted by a provider, they are more open to reflecting on their actions and beliefs — and may be more open to alternatives. Parents may ultimately change their behaviors, but only if the change becomes meaningful to them.

A frustration inherent in the relationship-based model of support is that parents may not change their behaviors, or may not change them enough for providers to feel that their efforts have made a difference. This is the nature of voluntary programs. Providers need not lose sight of their own goals for supporting parents based on their training, experience and knowledge of evidence-based best practices. In fact, letting families know the expectations of the program is a key element in the development of mutually respectful partnerships. But neither should providers assume that families are passive vessels for program goals. There may be a wide gulf between program goals (and the best practices as held by developmental and health experts) and the ideas and beliefs held by families. Of course, providers must also be aware that the research is not always clear on the best practices around feeding (eg, whether toddlers should be fed on regular schedules or allowed to graze).[25]

Because of these tensions, ongoing training and supervision of the frontline staff in early childhood intervention programs are critical. This is true for work with families in general, as well as for specific issues, such as early feeding practices. It is easy to memorize developmental milestones for eating and nutrition, use curriculum materials and handouts, and provide recommendations from professional groups.[23,26] But these tools serve little purpose if providers are not actively thinking about how the tools are meaningful (or not) to the families they serve.

Acknowledgments

Work presented in this paper was supported in part by grants from the Irving B. Harris Foundation to Jon Korfmacher (Erikson Institute) and the Maternal and Child Health Bureau (R40 MC 00203-04) to Sydney Hans (University of Chicago). Special thanks to Marisha Humphries and Xiaoli Wen for their contributions to the study results presented here.

References

1. Hulbert A. *Raising America: Experts, Parents, and a Century of Advice About Children.* New York, NY: Knopf Publishing; 2003.
2. Halpern R, Korfmacher J, Hilligoss E. *Parent Support and Education: Past History, Future Prospects* (Applied Research in Child Development, No. 6). Chicago, Ill: Erikson Institute; 2004.
3. National Research Council and Institute of Medicine, Committee on Integrating the Science of Early Childhood Development, Board on Children, Youth and Families, Commission on Behavioral and Social Sciences and Education. In: Shonkoff JP, Phillips DA, Keilty B, eds. *Early Childhood Intervention: Views From the Field (Report of a Workshop).* Washington, DC: National Academy Press; 2000.
4. Glink P. The Chicago Doula Project: a collaborative effort in perinatal support for birthing teens. *Zero to Three.* 1998;18(4):44-50.
5. Love JM, Kisker EE, Ross C, et al. The effectiveness of Early Head Start for 3-year-old children and their parents: lessons for policy and programs. *Developmental Psychology.* 2005;41:885-901.
6. Daro DA, Harding KA. Healthy Families America: using research to enhance practice. *Future of Children.* 1999;9(1):152-223.
7. Minkovitz CS, Hughart N, Strobino D, et al. A practice-based intervention to enhance quality of care in the first 3 years of life: the Healthy Steps for Young Children program. *Journal of the American Medical Association.* 2003;290:3081-3091.
8. Olds DL. The Nurse-Family Partnership: an evidence-based preventive intervention. *Infant Mental Health Journal.* 2006;27:5-25.
9. Wagner M, Spiker D, Linn MI. The effectiveness of the Parents as Teachers program with low-income parents and children. *Topics in Early Childhood Special Education.* 2002;22(2):67-81.
10. Karoly LA, Greenwood PW, Everingham SS, et al. *Investing in Our Children: What We Know and Don't Know About the Costs and Benefits of Early Childhood Interventions.* Santa Monica, Calif: RAND; 1998.
11. Olds D, Henderson CR Jr, Cole R, et al. Long-term effects of nurse home visitation on children's criminal and antisocial behavior: 15-year follow-up of a randomized controlled trial. *Journal of the American Medical Association.* 1998;280:1238-1244.
12. Sweet M, Appelbaum M. Is home visiting an effective strategy? A meta-analytic review of home visiting programs for families with young children. *Child Development.* 2004;75:1435-1456.
13. Emde RN, Korfmacher J, Kubicek LF. Towards a theory of early relationship-based intervention. In: Osofsky JD, Fitzgerald HI, eds. *World Association of Infant Mental Health Handbook of Infant Mental Health, Vol. 2: Early Intervention, Evaluation, & Assessment.* New York, NY: John Wiley & Sons; 2000.
14. Korfmacher J, Marchi I. The helping relationship in a teen parenting program. *Zero to Three.* 2002;23(2):21-26.
15. Florida State University Center for Prevention and Early Intervention Policy. *Partners for a Healthy Baby Home Visiting Curriculum.* Tallahassee, Fla: Florida State University; 2004.

16. Prevention Research Center for Family and Child Health. *Nurse-Family Partnership: Helping First-Time Parents Succeed.* Denver, Colo: University of Colorado Health Sciences Center; 2000.
17. Coveney J. What does research on families and food tell us? Implications for nutrition and dietetic practice. *Nutrition and Dietetics.* 2005;59:113-119.
18. Musick J, Stott F. Paraprofessionals revisited and reconsidered. In: Shonkoff JP, Meisels SJ, eds. *Handbook of Early Childhood Intervention.* 2nd ed. Cambridge, England: Cambridge University Press; 2000.
19. Klaus MH, Kennell JH, Klaus PH. *The Doula Book: How a Trained Labor Companion Can Help You Have a Shorter, Easier, and Healthier Birth.* 2nd ed. Cambridge, Mass: Da Capo Press; 2002.
20. Hans S. *Doula Support for Young Mothers: A Randomized Trial.* Final report to the Maternal and Child Health Bureau Research Program, R40 MC 00203-04. Washington, DC: Health Resources and Services Administration, Department of Health and Human Services; 2005.
21. Wambach KA, Koehn M. Experiences of infant-feeding decision-making among urban economically disadvantaged pregnant adolescents. *Journal of Advanced Nursing.* 2004;48:361-370.
22. Hans S, Korfmacher J. The professional development of paraprofessionals. *Zero to Three.* 2002; 23(2):4-8.
23. American Academy of Pediatrics. Breastfeeding and the use of human milk. *Pediatrics.* 2005; 115:496-506.
24. Bernstein V. Strengthening families through strengthening relationships: supporting the parent-child relationship through home visiting. *IMPrint: Newsletter of the Infant Mental Health Promotion Project.* Winter 2002-2003;35:2-6.
25. Lumeng J. What can we do to prevent childhood obesity? *Zero to Three.* 2005;25(3):13-19.
26. Gidding SS, Dennison BA, Birch LL, et al. Dietary recommendations for children and adolescents: a guide for practitioners. Consensus statement from the American Heart Association. *Circulation.* 2005;112:2061-2075.

Motivational Interviewing for Pediatric Obesity: Conceptual Issues and Evidence Review

Ken Resnicow, PhD
Rachel Davis, MPH
Stephen Rollnick, PhD

Introduction

Obesity and its medical and economic sequelae have risen dramatically among America's youth over the past 30 years.[1-4] Although ameliorating childhood obesity in the United States will require concerted effort at multiple levels of intervention, counseling by healthcare professionals represents an important component of the pubic health response. However, there are formidable barriers to counseling overweight children among pediatric practitioners, and, as a result, both the efficacy and reach of clinical interventions have been substantially limited.

Pediatric healthcare practitioners report low confidence in their ability to counsel overweight children or adolescents, and they also question the efficacy of behavioral counseling.[5-7] In one study,[5] for example, only 30% of pediatricians felt their efficacy for obesity counseling was "good to excellent," and only 10% felt obesity counseling was effective. In another study,[8] only 26% of pediatricians felt "quite" to "extremely" competent to counsel overweight youth, and only 37% felt "quite" to "extremely" comfortable providing such treatment. Almost 80% of pediatricians report feeling "very frustrated" treating pediatric obesity.[8] Low practitioner confidence and perceptions of treatment futility might stem from frustration over what practitioners perceive as low patient motivation and poor behavioral adherence.[5,6] Perceived patient indifference likely decreases practitioner efficacy as well as perceived treatment utility, which act synergistically to discourage practitioners from attempting to intervene. Importantly, these factors appear to be even more cogent inhibitors than lack of time or reimbursement, and they might be more amenable to intervention. Yet, despite low confidence in their counseling abilities, pediatricians and food and nutrition professionals are interested in improving their behavioral skills.[6,7]

One promising approach to weight-control counseling that might address both clinician confidence and treatment efficacy is motivational interviewing. As originally described by Miller[9] and more fully discussed in a seminal text by Miller and Rollnick,[10] motivational interviewing has been used extensively in the addiction field.[9,11-13] Numerous randomized trials have demonstrated its clinical efficacy for addictive behaviors.[14,15] Over the past 10 years, there has been considerable interest from public health, medical and dietetics practitioners in adapting motivational interviewing to address various chronic disease behaviors.[15-25] Although motivational interviewing has been used to modify diet and physical activity behaviors in adults, the evidence base for obesity prevention and treatment in children is just beginning to emerge.

This review will explore conceptual issues related to the application of motivational interviewing for the prevention and treatment of pediatric obesity. Given the paucity of studies on motivational interviewing and pediatric obesity, we will examine what is known about the application of motivational interviewing to modify diet and activity behaviors in children, adolescents and adults. We begin with a brief overview of motivational interviewing and describe some nuances of applying this approach to pediatric overweight.

Overview of Motivational Interviewing

Motivational interviewing is an egalitarian, empathetic "way of being" that manifests through specific techniques and strategies, such as reflective listening, shared decision making and agenda setting. One of the goals of motivational interviewing is to assist individuals in working through their ambivalence about behavior change. Motivational interviewing appears to be particularly effective for individuals who are initially less ready to change.[10,12,24,26,27] The tone of motivational interviewing is nonjudgmental, empathetic and encouraging. Counselors establish a nonconfrontational and supportive climate in which clients feel comfortable expressing both the positive and negative aspects of their current behavior. Ambivalence is fully explored and at least partially resolved prior to moving toward change. Many counseling models rely heavily on therapist insight, whereas traditional patient and nutrition education emphasize information exchange. In contrast, a motivational interviewing approach requires patients themselves to do much of the psychological work. A motivational interviewing counselor generally makes no direct attempt to dismantle denial, confront irrational or maladaptive beliefs, or convince or persuade. Instead, the counselor helps clients think about and verbally express their own reasons for and against change, and how their current behavior or health status affects their ability to achieve their life goals or fulfill core values. Motivational interviewing encourages clients to make fully informed and deeply contemplated life choices, even if the decision is not to change.

Motivational interviewing assumes that behavior change is affected more by motivation than information. Whereas the essence of motivational interviewing lies in its spirit, there are specific techniques and strategies that, when used effectively, help ensure that such a spirit is evoked. To achieve these ends, motivational interviewing counselors rely heavily on reflective listening and positive affirmations. Other core motivational interviewing techniques include allowing the client to interpret information, setting an agenda, rolling with resistance, building discrepancy and eliciting "change talk." As noted recently by Rollnick and colleagues,[28] motivational interviewing can be considered a form of guiding, as opposed to more directive methods that focus on advice and persuasion.

Reflective listening can be conceptualized as a form of hypothesis testing. The hypothesis can be stated in generic terms as, "If I heard you correctly, this is what I think you are saying...." or "Where you are going with this...." Reflections, particularly by counselors who are new to the technique, often begin with the phrase, "It sounds like...." More skilled counselors often phrase their reflections as more direct statements such as "You are having trouble with...", leaving off the assumed "It sounds like...." The goals of reflecting include demonstrating that the counselor has heard and is trying to understand the client, affirming the client's thoughts and feelings, and helping the client continue the process of self-discovery. One of the most important elements of mastering motivational interviewing is suppressing the instinct to respond with questions or advice. Questions can be biased by what the counselor may be interested in hearing about rather than what the client wants or needs to explore. Reflecting helps ensure that the direction of the encounter remains client-driven.

Reflections involve several levels of complexity or depth.[29] The simplest level tests whether the counselor understood the content of the client's statement. Deeper levels of reflection explore the meaning or feeling behind what was said. Effective deeper-level reflections can be thought of as the next sentence or next paragraph in the story (ie, "where the client is going with it"). A high level of reflective listening involves selectively reinforcing positive change talk that might be embedded in a litany of barriers. Similarly, skilled motivational interviewing counselors selectively reflect statements that build efficacy by focusing on prior successful efforts or reframing past unsuccessful attempts as practice rather than failure.

In standard medical and dietetics practice, practitioners often provide information about the risks of continuing a behavior or the benefits of change with the intent of persuasion. With regard to the parent of an overweight child, a traditional counseling statement might be, "It is very important that your child get control of his/her weight now before it becomes a bigger problem." In this style of communication, the practitioner often attempts to "push" motivation by increasing perceived risk. In contrast, information is discussed through motivational interviewing by first *eliciting* the person's understanding and information needs, then *providing* new information in a more neutral manner, followed by *eliciting* what this means for them with a question like, "How do you make sense of all this?" Motivational interviewing practitioners avoid persuasion with "predigested" health messages and instead allow clients to process information and find their own personal relevance. To this end, the guideline "elicit-provide-elicit" has been proposed as a framework for exchanging information in the spirit of motivational interviewing.

Confronting clients can lead to defensiveness, rapport breakage and, ultimately, poor outcomes.[9] Therefore, motivational interviewing counselors avoid argumentation and instead "roll with resistance." A motivational interviewing encounter resembles a dance more than a wrestling match.[30] For example, a parent might raise doubts that their child's weight is a problem or suggest that the child's weight will improve on its own as the child ages. Rather than stating facts to counter such beliefs, a motivational interviewing practitioner would reflect the parent's doubt and then provide opportunities for the parent to voice any concerns they might have about the child remaining overweight or gaining weight. In cases where a parent's resistance is severe, the practitioner might use an amplified negative reflection, such as "It appears that you see no real problem with your child's weight" or "Having your child watch TV most of the afternoon really works for you and your family." This potentially risky strategy is designed to "unstick" the entrenched client by short-circuiting the "yes-but" cycle.

A core principle of motivational interviewing is that individuals are more likely to accept and act upon those opinions and plans that they voice themselves.[31] The more a person argues for a position, the greater his or her commitment to it often becomes. Therefore, clients are encouraged to express their own reasons and plans for change (or lack thereof). This process is referred to as eliciting change talk. One technique to elicit change talk is the use of importance/confidence rulers.[26,30,32] This strategy begins with 2 questions: (a) "On a scale from 0 to 10, with 10 being the highest, how important is it to you to change your child's/family's (insert target behavior)?" and (b) "On a scale from 0 to 10, with 10 being the highest, assuming you wanted to change this behavior in your child/family, how confident are you that you could (insert target behavior)?" These 2 questions assess the client's importance and confidence for change, respectively.[11,32] Clinicians follow each of these questions with 2 probes. If the client answered "5," for example, the counselor would probe first with "Why did you not choose a lower number, like a 3 or a 4?" followed by "What would it take to get you to a 6 or a 7?" These probes elicit positive change talk and ideas for potential solutions from the client.

To help parents establish discrepancy between their child's/family's current behavior and their personal core values or life goals, our group has developed a values list tailored to parents of overweight youth (see Figure 1) that is used to identify what is important to parents about their children and families. Practitioners then probe parents to see if they can find any connections between their child's weight behaviors and the values they selected.

Figure 1. Values list for counseling parents of overweight children used in the Healthy Lifestyles Pilot Study.

Values for your child	Values for you	Values for your family
Be healthy	Good parent	Cohesive
Be strong	Responsible	Healthy
Have many friends	Disciplined	Peaceful meals
Be fit	Good spouse	Getting along
Have high self-esteem	Respected at home	Spending time together
Not being teased	On top of things	Be able to communicate feelings
Not feeling left out	Spiritual	Fulfill our potential

Three Communication Styles: A Route to Integration

It can be challenging for practitioners to fit motivational interviewing into their everyday practice. Some view it as a highly specialized skill that is difficult for the typical physician to effectively integrate and is preferentially delivered by psychologists. Yet, it is also striking how brief consultations by skilled physicians can approach the spirit and even the "laws" of motivational interviewing. One resolution to this "intimidation factor" proposed by Rollnick and colleagues[28] is to place motivational interviewing within a model of communication that comprises 3 naturally occurring communication styles: directing, guiding and following. When practitioners use a directing style, they primarily inform patients about what they think the patients should do and why they should do it. This is similar to what is often referred to as anticipatory guidance. Conversely, when practitioners use a more guiding style, they rely less on persuasion and instead encourage patients to explore their motivations and aspirations. Following involves understanding and tracking the patient's story, and is typically used in the early phase of a consultation and under special circumstances, such as when responding to a bereaved individual.

Skillfulness is defined as the ability to move flexibly between these styles according to patient needs. The guiding style is seen as particularly suited to consultations involving health behavior change, and motivational interviewing is defined as a refined form of this naturally occurring guiding style. Seen in this light, the task for practitioners in the pediatric obesity field is to improve their guiding abilities while suppressing the instinct to direct.

Applying Motivational Interviewing to Pediatric Obesity: Conceptual and Pragmatic Issues

There are several aspects of obesity counseling for children and adolescents that pose unique challenges for the motivational interviewing practitioner. First, depending on the age of the patient, the intervention can occur directly with the parent(s), directly with the child or with both parent(s) and child. There is some evidence that older obese children do not benefit from involvement of their parents, whereas parent involvement can be beneficial for younger children.[33] However, it is not known at what age youth and parents should be seen alone versus together. In addition, a general issue regarding use of motivational interviewing with children is that practitioners might need to use more questions as opposed to reflections in order to elicit responses.

Secondly, obesity is not a behavior per se. Therefore, a key task for clinicians is to work with parents and/or youth to identify what behaviors contribute to the child's weight status and use agenda-setting strategies to determine which behaviors they feel are most amenable to intervention. Although motivational interviewing has been established as a useful method for helping individuals overcome resistance and clarify motivation, it is important to note that additional strategies, such as behavior therapy[34] or cognitive behavioral therapy,[35] might be needed once an individual decides to attempt behavior change. There is a motivational interviewing-consistent means for delivering such treatment and, at this stage of care, motivational interviewing should perhaps be conceived as a platform for treatment delivery rather than the primary treatment modality. How to best integrate standard cognitive and behavioral weight-loss strategies from a training and clinical perspective merits examination.

Identification of Prior Studies Using Motivational Interviewing

Studies were identified by electronic search of the MEDLINE database using various combinations of key search terms, including *motivational interviewing, motivational enhancement, obesity, children, adolescents, nutrition, diet* and *physical activity.* Additional studies were identified through bibliographies of published studies and informal communication with peers. Given the lack of published randomized trials of motivational interviewing for treatment or prevention of pediatric obesity, we decided to include in our review pediatric obesity pilot studies, youth studies where motivational interviewing was used to modify diet or physical activity, youth studies on diabetes, adult studies of motivational interviewing to modify diet or physical activity, and studies addressing the use of motivational interviewing to modify other behaviors in children and adolescents, which almost exclusively involved substance use.

Motivational Interviewing Studies Targeting Pediatric Obesity

We identified only 2 studies in which motivational interviewing was used to intervene on pediatric obesity (Table 1). The first of these studies, the Healthy Lifestyles Pilot Study (Dietz and colleagues, unpublished data, 2005), focused on prevention of overweight among children 3 to 7 years old. The second study, Go Girls, was a multicomponent intervention for overweight African-American adolescents aged 12 to 16 years, which included motivational interviewing as a key intervention element.

Healthy Lifestyles Pilot Study

The Healthy Lifestyles Pilot Study was conducted from 2004 to 2005 as a partnership of the Centers for Disease Control and Prevention, the American Academy of Pediatrics and the American Dietetic Association. The primary aim of the Healthy Lifestyles Pilot Study was to examine the feasibility and potential efficacy of pediatrician and registered dietitian (RD) motivational interviewing counseling for preventing childhood obesity in primary care pediatrics. Study sites were members of the American Academy of Pediatrics Pediatric Research in Office Settings Network, which is a practice-based

Table 1. Studies Using Motivational Interviewing for Control of Pediatric Weight, Diet and Physical Activity

Study	Starting number	Age (y)	Outcome/ design	Intervention	Interventionist
Healthy Lifestyles, Dietz and colleagues (unpublished), 2005	93	3-7	BMI[a] Pilot	Standard care Moderate = 1 MI[b] (MD[c]) High = 2 MI (MD)+2 MI (RD[d])	Pediatricians Dietitians
Go Girls, Resnicow and colleagues, 2005[37]	147	12-16	BMI RCT[e]	Multicomponent Group session and 4-6 phone MI	Health educators Psychologists
DISC,[f] Berg-Smith and colleagues, 1999[21]	127	13-17	Diet Lipids No control	1 in person MI 1 phone MI	Health educators Dietitians
Channon and colleagues, 2003[38]	40	14-18	HbA1c[g] Nonparticipants as controls	Variable 1-9 mean 4.7	Investigator
Knight and colleagues, 2003[39]	20	13-16	Perceptions about DM[h]	Six 1-hr sessions Qualitative response	Registered nurse Senior registrar

[a]BMI = body mass index; calculated as kg/m²
[b]MI = motivational interviewing
[c]MD = physician
[d]RD = registered dietitian
[e]RCT = randomized controlled trial
[f]DISC = Dietary Intervention Study in Children
[g]HbA1c = hemoglobin A1c
[h]DM = diabetes mellitus

research network established by the American Academy of Pediatrics in 1986.[36] Fifteen Pediatric Research in Office Settings practices were assigned by the investigators to 1 of 3 conditions: control, minimal intervention or intensive intervention. Five practices were allocated to each arm. The intervention phase lasted 6 months. Each of the 15 Pediatric Research in Office Settings practices was asked to recruit 10 patients. Subject eligibility included children ages 3 to 7 years with either a body mass index (BMI; calculated at kg/m^2) for age and sex between the 85th and 95th percentiles or a combination of at least 1 parent with a BMI >30 and a BMI for age and sex between the 50th and 85th percentiles. Parents in all groups completed questionnaires at baseline and again 6 months later (Table 2).

Table 2. Parent Perceptions of Pediatrician and Dietitian Motivational Interviewing in the Healthy Lifestyles Pilot Study (n = 16)

Questionnaire Item	**% of Parents Agreeing "A Lot"**
My pediatrician listened to me	100
My pediatrician asked my opinion about things	88
My pediatrician asked permission before giving me information or advice	88
My pediatrician helped me think about why changing my family's food habits is important	94
My pediatrician was supportive/encouraging	94
My pediatrician discussed values that were important to me	88
My pediatrician helped me think about why changing my family's television-viewing habits is important	63
The nutritionist listened to me	100
The nutritionist asked my opinion about things	100
The nutritionist asked permission before giving me information or advice	88
The nutritionist helped me think about why changing my family's food habits is important	100
The nutritionist was supportive/encouraging	100
The nutritionist discussed values that were important to me	88
The nutritionist helped me think about why changing my family's television-viewing habits is important	50

The only intervention provided to participants in the control group consisted of 2 safety education tip sheets. Parents of children in the minimal-intervention group received a single, brief motivational interviewing counseling session from their pediatrician 1 month after baseline. Pediatricians in the minimal intervention group were trained to provide counseling in a 2-day motivational interviewing workshop. In contrast, participants in the intensive-intervention group engaged in 4 motivational interviewing counseling sessions. Two sessions were led by the patient's pediatrician, and 2 sessions were guided by an RD. These counseling sessions were delivered at 1 month and 3 months postenrollment.

Physicians and RDs were trained at a joint, 2-day motivational interviewing workshop. The RD-led sessions were longer than those with the pediatricians, generally in the range of 30 to 45 minutes. Sick visits continued as usual for children in both groups. Recruitment occurred from April through November 2004. One minimal intervention practice dropped out, leaving a total of 93 enrolled patients from 14 practices.

To assess competence in motivational interviewing skill, clinicians participating in the Healthy Lifestyles Pilot Study completed a measure of motivational interviewing fidelity developed by the Healthy Lifestyles Pilot Study investigators called the 1-PASS. The 1-PASS consists of self-evaluation rating forms on which performance on several motivational interviewing dimensions is scored on a scale of 1 to 7. Scores of 4.0 and higher are considered an indication of adequate motivational interviewing proficiency. Using audiotapes of the Healthy Lifestyles Pilot Study intervention encounters, a trained psychologist rated each motivational interviewing session using 1-PASS and then discussed the score with each clinician. Overall scores for the first patient encounters ranged from 3.2 for moderate-intensity pediatricians to 4.4 for high-intensity intervention group RDs. Overall scores were slightly higher in the second encounters, ranging from 3.7 to 5.8 for pediatricians and RDs combined. For the 6 clinicians who participated in 2 supervisor feedback sessions, mean motivational interviewing skills scores increased 1.1 points between the first and second encounters. Outcomes of the Healthy Lifestyles Pilot Study on BMI and self-reported behavior are forthcoming (R. Schwartz, Wake Forest University School of Medicine, Winston-Salem, NC, unpublished data, 2006). Process results indicate that parents reported high satisfaction with the counseling from the pediatricians and RDs.

Go Girls

Go Girls was a church-based nutrition and physical activity program designed for overweight African-American adolescent females.[37] Ten predominantly middle socioeconomic status churches were randomized to either a high-intensity (20 to 26 sessions) or moderate-intensity (6 sessions) culturally tailored behavioral group intervention delivered over 6 months. Each session included an experiential behavioral activity, approximately 30 minutes of physical activity, and preparation and tasting of healthy foods. In the high-intensity group, girls also received 4 to 6 motivational interviewing telephone counseling calls. Counselors were either health educators with master's degrees or doctorate-trained psychologists. All counselors received 2 days of experiential motivational interviewing training by the first author (Resnicow), plus ongoing clinical supervision by doctoral-level psychologists. Telephone calls were synchronized with the group sessions to ensure that the motivational interviewing calls focused on participants' plans and progress regarding the same topics covered during each weekly group session. Calls lasted approximately 20 to 30 minutes each, and were generally conducted in the afternoon or evening.

From the 10 churches, 123 girls completed the baseline and 6-month follow-up assessments. The primary outcome was BMI. The 6-month assessments indicated a net difference of 0.5 BMI units between the high and moderate intensity. This difference was not statistically significant ($P = .20$). In addition, there was no association between change in BMI and the number of motivational interviewing calls completed in the high-intensity group. An additional follow-up assessment was conducted at 1 year postbaseline, and findings mirrored those found at 6 months.

Motivational Interviewing Studies Addressing Dyslipidemia and Diabetes

Dietary Intervention Study in Children

The Dietary Intervention Study in Children was a multicenter, randomized controlled trial sponsored by the National Heart, Lung, and Blood Institute to assess the efficacy of dietary counseling to decrease elevated serum lipids (low-density lipoprotein cholesterol).[21] Children with elevated low-density lipoprotein cholesterol entered the initial clinical trial when they were 8 to

10 years of age. As the intervention cohort moved into adolescence, the investigators elected to add a motivational interviewing-based intervention to "renew" adherence to the prescribed diet among the original intervention group (there was no control group for this phase). The counselors were primarily master's-level health educators and RDs who received 18 hours of motivational interviewing training. Each study participant received 1 in-person motivational interviewing session and 1 follow-up session that was conducted either in person or by telephone. Twenty-four-hour recall data from the first 127 youths to complete the 2-session protocol indicated that the proportion of calories from fat and dietary cholesterol was substantially reduced at the 3-month follow-up assessment. Mean proportion of calories from fat decreased from 27.7% to 25.6% ($P<.001$), and overall dietary adherence scores improved. When asked about their reaction to the counseling, 74% of the youths reported being satisfied or very satisfied.

Other Studies Targeting Diabetes

In a pilot study, Channon and colleagues[38] tested the impact of motivational interviewing on 22 adolescents, 14 to 18 years of age, with diabetes.[38] Participating youth received between 1 and 9 motivational interviewing sessions each, with an average of 4.7 sessions over 6 months. The focus of the motivational interviewing sessions consisted of awareness building (analyzing pros and cons), finding alternatives, problem solving, goal setting and minimizing confrontation. Between 8 weeks and 6 months after the end of the intervention phase, patients who had received motivational interviewing showed a substantial reduction in hemoglobin A1c from an average baseline measure of 10.8% to approximately 10.0%.

Knight and colleagues[39] administered a motivational interviewing-based group intervention in 6 weekly, 1-hour sessions to 6 youth 13 to 16 years of age with poorly controlled type 1 diabetes mellitus. The intervention included externalizing conversations, as well as motivational interviewing. Participation in the motivational interviewing-based group was compared with a "usual care" control group (n = 14). At the 6-month follow-up assessment, adolescents who had received the group motivational interviewing were more likely than those youth in the control group to display positive shifts in their perception of diabetes, such as increased feelings of control and acceptance. Changes in behavior or physiologic outcomes were not assessed.

Studies on Diet and Physical Activity Among Adults

We identified 8 controlled-outcome studies and 1 pilot study where motivational interviewing was used to modify diet and/or physical activity in adults.[22,24,40-48] In none of these studies was weight the primary target. With the exception of the studies by Mhurchu and colleagues[40] and Woollard and colleagues,[47,48] each study showed a substantial effect favoring the motivational interviewing group on at least 1 main outcome. In all 3 studies where motivational interviewing was used to modify fruit and vegetable intake, substantial effects were observed. In the 4 studies where weight was at least a secondary target outcome, only 1, Woollard and colleagues,[41] found a considerable effect. Although Harland and colleagues[42] found a short-term effect of motivational interviewing on physical activity, substantial long-term outcomes in this study and the Healthy Body/Healthy Spirit[46] study were not observed. In those studies where motivational interviewing showed important outcomes, effect sizes were generally in the small-to-moderate range, 0.20 to 0.50, as defined by Cohen.[49]

Studies of Motivational Interviewing for Other Adolescent Behaviors

Motivational interviewing has also been used in studies with adolescent smokers. In a pilot study, Colby and colleagues[16] compared motivational interviewing with brief advice in a study of 40 adolescent smokers recruited from a single hospital who were seeking care for conditions generally unrelated to smoking. Participants in the motivational interviewing group viewed 4 videotaped vignettes aimed to stimulate discussion. At the follow-up assessment, 20% reported 7-day smoking abstinence in the motivational interviewing group compared with 10% in the brief advice group. In the motivational interviewing group, 72% made a quit attempt versus 60% in the advice group. These differences were not statistically significant, possibly because of the small sample size employed.

In a subsequent study, the same researchers evaluated the efficacy of using a brief motivational interviewing intervention with adolescents from a hospital outpatient clinic or emergency department.[50] Patients 14 to 19 years of age who were not seeking treatment for smoking were proactively screened and recruited. The motivational interviewing counselors were 7 bachelor's to master's-level staff with 1 to 4 years of clinical counseling experience. Training included reading assignments, 40 hours of experiential workshops and weekly group supervision. Patients were randomly assigned to receive either one session of motivational interviewing or standardized brief advice to quit smoking. The former generally lasted 35 minutes and the latter about 5 minutes. Both groups received a brief follow-up telephone contact 1 week later. The final sample consisted of 25 males and 60 females with an average age of 16.3 years. At 1-month and 3-month postenrollment, there were no significant between-group differences in self-reported 7-day abstinence or biochemically validated quitting. At 6 months, there was a significant effect ($P<.05$) favoring the motivational interviewing group in self-reported quitting compared to the brief advice group, at 23% and 3%, respectively. However, the differences based on the biochemically confirmed rates, 9% vs 2%, were not statistically significant.

Future Research Questions

The studies reviewed here indicate that motivational interviewing might be feasible with children and adolescents. However, there are insufficient data to determine the efficacy of motivational interviewing for the prevention or treatment of pediatric obesity or other domains of behavior change in children. Data from adult studies suggest that motivational interviewing can be effective in modifying diet and at least short-term physical activity. However, direct evidence of efficacy for weight control in adults is lacking. It should be noted that none of the adult studies targeted weight as the primary outcome.

To establish the efficacy of motivational interviewing for pediatric and adult weight control, several methodologic issues will have to be addressed. First, it is important to address intervention fidelity. Failure to assess and statistically control for treatment fidelity can result in type III error. This occurs when negative or weak results are due to poor intervention delivery but are erroneously attributed to failure of the intervention itself. Few studies have provided evidence of counselor competence or fidelity to motivational interviewing. This is complicated by the fact that there is considerable variability in how motivational interviewing is conceptualized, executed and assessed across studies. There are no widely accepted criteria for what comprises a motivational interviewing intervention or for measuring how rigorously these components are administered.

An important question that should be examined is the extent to which the effects of motivational interviewing-informed interventions can be attributed to motivational interviewing per se, as opposed to more generic elements of counseling such as attention effects and empathy. A related problem is that in several positive studies, internal validity is threatened by the fact that the motivational interviewing interventions were often additive to other interventions. Client contact was often not comparable across conditions, as the comparison groups did not receive any "sham" or alternative counseling. Determining the efficacy of motivational interviewing with high internal validity can be achieved by comparing motivational interviewing head-to-head with other counseling methods while holding intervention intensity, duration and delivery modality constant. An example of this is Project MATCH.[13] An important issue for pediatric obesity is determining the appropriate age at which to begin intervening directly with youth, as opposed to their parents, and when, if at all, parents should be included in the counseling.[33]

Tailoring Counseling Style to Different Client Needs and Preferences: It Is Not for Everyone

Although many patients report high satisfaction and improved outcomes from patient-centered communication approaches,[51-53] such as motivational interviewing, some individuals prefer a more directive, educational style.[54] Practitioners therefore need to tailor their intervention style to client needs, preferences and culture. Absent methods for triaging which style to employ for particular client subgroups, clinicians might need to test various techniques with each client and rely on clinical judgment to determine which approach best fits each client.

Challenge of Technology Transfer

Many of the strategies and programs recommended for medical management of obesity were developed and tested under efficacy conditions.[55,56] Under these circumstances, interventions are generally delivered by highly skilled practitioners who typically receive extensive training and supervision. The extent to which research-based interventions can be replicated under real-world conditions, where clinicians might receive only brief in-service training and supervision, remains unclear. While the primary "gatekeepers" for detection and treatment of obesity appear to be primary care physicians, many (if not most) previously successful interventions were conducted by psychologists or behavioral specialists. This is also true for motivational interviewing interventions, where counselors were usually highly trained behavioral specialists. More research is needed to develop and test motivational interviewing-based interventions that a priori are designed for delivery by pediatric practitioners and account for limitations in medical training, as well as the field's implicit "disease" orientation, practice structure and reimbursement guidelines.

Recast Obesity as a Cluster of Heterogeneous Conditions: Consider the Obesities

Perhaps like cancer, obesity should be considered not as 1 disease but a rubric of many diseases, each with a unique etiology, course and treatment. As noted by Epstein and colleagues,[57] "Treating obesity as a homogenous condition, with all participants receiving a common intervention, might contribute to the mixed treatment outcomes that are reported." Factors operative in obesity include: age, sex, dietary patterns, physical activity, socioeconomics, psychosocial issues, metabolism, comorbidities, familial/genetic determinants and racial/ethnic/cultural characteristics. With each of these factors having a greater or lesser influence on obesity in any individual case, classification and subclassification schemes should be developed to adequately describe the heterogeneity of the obesities.

The reasons for energy imbalance in children can be highly variable across individuals, and treatment programs can be better tailored to these individual differences. For example, excess caloric intake could result from consuming high-fat foods or foods high in simple carbohydrates. For some high-fat food consumers, excess caloric intake could be attributed to 1 or 2 foods, while for others excess intake could be attributed to a variety of foods.

In addition to focusing on specific foods, tailoring could also account for eating patterns, such as consuming large serving sizes, rapid eating, eating second helpings or eating at "all you can eat" establishments. Factors related to physical inactivity are likely to be equally individualistic, providing a similar rationale for tailoring treatment. However, despite numerous potential differences in behavioral patterns, our current detection and treatment algorithms often fail to account for such microlevel individual differences. An advantage of motivational interviewing is that its emphasis on "pulling" rather than "pushing" enables clinicians to better tailor interventions to the behavioral and psychologic needs of their clients.

Implications for Practitioners

Although the efficacy and cost-effectiveness of motivational interviewing for the prevention or treatment of pediatric obesity have not yet been clearly established, evidence from motivational interviewing for other health concerns combined with the considerable research on client-centered communication can be sufficient to encourage food and nutrition professionals to consider obtaining training in motivational interviewing and to begin incorporating these techniques into their practice. The American Dietetic Association has, in fact, begun to offer motivational interviewing workshops at both national and regional American Dietetic Association meetings. While motivational interviewing appears useful for helping clients resolve ambivalence and solidify motivation, clinicians might also require behavioral skills to employ during the "action" phase of treatment. Such treatment, however, should be generally delivered in a client-centered style. In recognition that some parents and youth might respond better to more directive counseling than a motivational interviewing style, clinicians should tailor their intervention approaches to their clients' needs.

Conclusions

Ultimately, the essential question might not be whether motivational interviewing is effective for control of pediatric obesity but how effective, in what populations, at what dose and at what cost. Which pediatric healthcare providers are best able to deliver motivational interviewing with sufficient fidelity, how much training is needed to raise their competence to adequate levels, and how best to impart clinical skills at various career stages should also be explored. How different healthcare delivery systems might be willing and able to incorporate motivational interviewing into training and clinical guidelines and how pediatric healthcare providers are reimbursed for training and delivery of motivational interviewing also merit examination.

References

1. Finkelstein E, Fiebelkorn I, Wang G. National medical spending attributable to overweight and obesity: how much, and who's paying? *Health Affairs.* 2003;W3:219-226.
2. Wolf A, Colditz GA. Current estimates of the economic cost of obesity in the United States. *Obesity Research.* 1998;6:97-106.
3. Must A, Spadano J, Coakley EH, Field AE, Colditz G, Dietz WH. The disease burden associated with overweight and obesity. *Journal of the American Medical Association.* 1999;282:1523-1529.
4. Dietz W. Health consequences of obesity in youth: childhood predictors of adult disease. *Pediatrics.* 1998;101(suppl 3):518-525.
5. Kolagotla L, Adams W. Ambulatory management of childhood obesity. *Obesity Research.* 2004;12: 275-283.
6. Story MT, Neumark-Stzainer DR, Sherwood NE, et al. Management of child and adolescent obesity: attitudes, barriers, skills, and training needs among healthcare professionals. *Pediatrics.* 2002;110:210-214.
7. Perrin EM, Flower KB, Garrett J, Ammerman AS. Preventing and treating obesity: pediatricians' self-efficacy, barriers, resources, and advocacy. *Ambulatory Pediatrics.* 2005;5:150-156.
8. Jelalian E, Boergers J, Alday CS, Frank R. Survey of physician attitudes and practices related to pediatric obesity. *Clinical Pediatrics.* 2003;42:235-245.
9. Miller WR. Motivational interviewing with problem drinkers. *Behavioural Psychotherapy.* 1983; 11:147-172.
10. Miller W, Rollnick S. *Motivational Interviewing: Preparing People to Change Addictive Behavior.* New York, NY: Guilford Press; 1991.
11. Rollnick S, Heather N, Gold R, Hall W. Development of a short "readiness to change" questionnaire for use in brief, opportunistic interventions among excessive drinkers. *British Journal of Addiction.* 1992;87:743-754.
12. Heather N, Rollnick S, Bell A, Richmond R. Effects of brief counselling among male heavy drinkers identified on general hospital wards. *Drug and Alcohol Review.* 1996;15:29-38.
13. Kadden RM. Project MATCH: treatment main effects and matching results. *Alcoholism, Clinical and Experimental Research.* 1996;20(suppl 8):196A-197A.
14. Burke BL, Arkowitz H, Menchola M. The efficacy of motivational interviewing: a meta-analysis of controlled clinical trials. *Journal of Consulting and Clinical Psychology.* 2003;71:843-861.
15. Dunn C, Deroo L, Rivara F. The use of brief interventions adapted from motivational interviewing across behavioral domains: a systematic review. *Addiction.* 2001;96:1725-1742.
16. Colby SM, Monti PM, Barnett NP, et al. Brief motivational interviewing in a hospital setting for adolescent smoking: a preliminary study. *Journal of Consulting and Clinical Psychology.* 1998;66: 574-578.
17. Ershoff DH, Quinn VP, Boyd NR, Stern J, Gregory M, Wirtschafter D. The Kaiser Permanente prenatal smoking cessation trial: when more isn't better, what is enough? *American Journal of Preventive Medicine.* 1999;17:161-168.
18. Stott NCH, Rollnick S, Pill RM. Innovation in clinical method: diabetes care and negotiating skills. *Family Practice.* 1995;12:413-418.
19. Miller WR. Motivational interviewing: research, practice, and puzzles. *Addictive Behaviors.* 1996; 21:835-842.
20. Velasquez M, Hecht J, Quinn V, Emmons K, DiClimente C, Dolan-Mullen P. Application of motivational interviewing to prenatal smoking cessation: training and implementation issues. *Tobacco Control.* 2000;9(suppl III):36-40.
21. Berg-Smith S, Stevens V, Brown K, et al. A brief motivational intervention to improve dietary adherence in adolescents. *Health Education Research.* 1999;14:399-410.

22. Smith D, Heckemeyer C, Kratt P, Mason D. Motivational interviewing to improve adherence to a behavioral weight-control program for older obese women with NIDDM. *Diabetes Care.* 1997; 20:52-54.
23. Emmons K, Rollnick S. Motivational interviewing in healthcare settings: opportunities and limitations. *American Journal of Preventive Medicine.* 2001;20:68-74.
24. Resnicow K, Jackson A, Wang T, Dudley W, Baranowski T. A motivational interviewing intervention to increase fruit and vegetable intake through black churches: results of the Eat for Life Trial. *American Journal of Public Health.* 2001;91:1686-1693.
25. Resnicow K, DiIorio C, Soet JE, Ernst D, Borrelli B, Hecht J. Motivational interviewing in health promotion: it sounds like something is changing. *Health Psychology.* 2002;21:444-451.
26. Butler C, Rollnick S, Cohen D, Bachman M, Russell I, Stott N. Motivational consulting versus brief advice for smokers in general practice: a randomized trial. *British Journal of General Practice.* 1999;49:611-616.
27. Rollnick S, Miller WR. What is motivational interviewing? *Behavioural and Cognitive Psychotherapy.* 1995;23:325-334.
28. Rollnick S, Butler C, Cambridge J, Kinnersley P, Elwyn G, Resnicow K. Consultations about behaviour change. *British Medical Journal.* 2005;331:961-963.
29. Carkhuff R. *The Art of Helping.* 7th ed. Amherst, Mass: Human Resource Development Press; 1993.
30. Rollnick S, Mason P, Butler C. *Health Behavior Change: A Guide for Practitioners.* London, UK: Churchill Livingstone (Harcourt Brace Inc); 1999.
31. Bem D. Self-perception theory. In: Berkowitz L, ed. *Advances in Experimental Social Psychology.* New York, NY: Academic Press; 1972:1-62.
32. Rollnick S, Butler CC, Stott N. Helping smokers make decisions: the enhancement of brief intervention for general medical practice. *Patient Education and Counseling.* 1997;31:191-203.
33. Resnicow K. Obesity prevention and treatment in youth: what is known? In: Trowbridge FL, Kibbe D, eds. *Childhood Obesity: Partnerships for Research and Prevention.* Washington, DC: ILSI Press; 2002:11-30.
34. Latner JD, Wilson GT, Stunkard AJ, Jackson ML. Self-help and long-term behavior therapy for obesity. *Behaviour Research and Therapy.* 2002;40:804-812.
35. Foreyt JP, Poston WS. What is the role of cognitive-behavior therapy in patient management? *Obesity Research.* 1998;6(suppl 1):18S-22S.
36. Wasserman R, Slora E, Bocian A, et al. Pediatric research in office settings (PROS): a national practice-based research network to improve children's healthcare. *Pediatrics.* 1998;102:1350-1357.
37. Resnicow K, Taylor R, Baskin M. Results of Go Girls: a nutrition and physical activity intervention for overweight African American adolescent females conducted through black churches. *Obesity Research.* 2005;13:1739-1748.
38. Channon S, Smith VJ, Gregory JW. A pilot study of motivational interviewing in adolescents with diabetes. *Archives of Disease in Childhood.* 2003;88:680-683.
39. Knight KM, Bundy C, Morris R, et al. The effects of group motivational interviewing and externalizing conversations for adolescents with type-1 diabetes. *Psychology, Health & Medicine.* 2003;8: 149-158.
40. Mhurchu CN, Margetts BM, Speller V. Randomized clinical trial comparing the effectiveness of two dietary interventions for patients with hyperlipidaemia. *Clinical Science.* 1998;95:479-487.
41. Woollard J, Beilin L, Lord T, Puddey I, MacAdam D, Rouse I. A controlled trial of nurse counselling on lifestyle change for hypertensives treated in general practice: preliminary results. *Clinical and Experimental Pharmacology & Physiology.* 1995;22:466-468.
42. Harland J, White M, Drinkwater C, Chinn D, Farr L, Howel D. The Newcastle exercise project: a randomised controlled trial of methods to promote physical activity in primary care. *British Medical Journal.* 1999;319:828-832.

43. Resnicow K, Coleman-Wallace D, Jackson A, et al. Dietary change through black churches: baseline results and program description of the Eat for Life Trial. *Journal of Cancer Education.* 2000;15:156-163.
44. Bowen D, Ehret C, Pedersen M, et al. Results of an adjunct dietary intervention program in the Women's Health Initiative. *Journal of the American Dietetic Association.* 2002;102:1631-1637.
45. Resnicow K, Campbell MK, Carr C, et al. Body and soul. A dietary intervention conducted through African-American churches. *American Journal of Preventive Medicine.* 2004;27:97-105.
46. Resnicow K, Jackson A, Blissett D, et al. Results of the Healthy Body Healthy Spirit Trial. *Health Psychology.* 2005;24: 339-348.
47. Woollard J, Burke V, Beilin LJ. Effects of general practice-based nurse-counselling on ambulatory blood pressure and antihypertensive drug prescription in patients at increased risk of cardiovascular disease. *Journal of Human Hypertension.* 2003;17:689-695.
48. Woollard J, Burke V, Beilin LJ, Verheijden M, Bulsara MK. Effects of a general practice-based intervention on diet, body mass index and blood lipids in patients at cardiovascular risk. *Journal of Cardiovascular Risk.* 2003;10:31-40.
49. Cohen J. A power primer. *Psychological Bulletin.* 1992;112:155-159.
50. Colby SM, Monti PM, Tevyaw TOL, et al. Brief motivational intervention for adolescent smokers in medical settings. *Addictive Behavior.* 2005;30:865-874.
51. Stewart MA. Effective physician-patient communication and health outcomes: a review. *Canadian Medical Association Journal.* 1995;152:1423-1433.
52. Wanzer MB, Booth-Butterfield M, Gruber K. Perceptions of healthcare providers' communication: relationships between patient-centered communication and satisfaction. *Health Communication.* 2004;16:363-383.
53. Roter DL, Hall JA. Physician gender and patient-centered communication: a critical review of empirical research. *Annual Review of Public Health.* 2004;25:497-519.
54. Swenson SL, Buell S, Zettler P, White M, Ruston DC, Lo B. Patient-centered communication: do patients really prefer it? *Journal of General Internal Medicine.* 2004;19:1069-1079.
55. Barlow SE, Dietz WH. Obesity evaluation and treatment: expert committee recommendations. The Maternal and Child Health Bureau, Health Resources and Services Administration and the Department of Health and Human Services. *Pediatrics.* 1998;102:e29.
56. NIH-NHLBI and the North American Association for the Study of Obesity. *The Practical Guide: Identification, Evaluation, and Treatment of Overweight and Obesity in Adults.* NIH Publication. No. 00-4084, 2000.
57. Epstein L, Myers M, Raynor H, Saelens B. Treatment of pediatric obesity. *Pediatrics.* 1998;101: 554-570.

Mealtimes and Beyond: Ways of Working With Parents When Eating Difficulties Prevail

Mary Rudolf, MB

"Tis time to shew the careful mother, when
To shut the fountains, and the child to wean.
But such the changing lot of man below,
That none, for this, a certain rule can know:
The best-laid plans oft most deceitful prove,
And fate and fortune all our hopes remove."

Scevole de Ste Marthe
Paedotrophia 1584

Introduction

The verse that opens this chapter is from an early parenting "manual." It was written by a French nobleman in the 16th century who had lost 2 sons to smallpox. When a third son fell ill and physicians were unable to help him, de Ste Marthe applied himself to find his own remedies. On the child's recovery he was entreated by friends to communicate his experience to the public. The result was a 3-volume didactic poem in Latin on pregnancy, the care of the infant and childhood illness.[1] It was dedicated to King Henri III, who decreed on its publication in 1584 that it should be translated into French "to the end that all France might have more particular understanding of this most learned and useful labour." More than 4 centuries later, parents, physicians, researchers and policymakers are focusing on the same subject, and perhaps can still learn from the poem. De Ste Marthe, in his wisdom, emphasises how fate and fortune can divert parents from following best-laid nutritional recommendations, and how emotionally devastating this can be.

As a paediatrician I have spent much of my career working with young children with failure to thrive, the majority of whom are difficult to feed. It is my contention that by studying these children, we can learn a great deal about young children's eating behaviour, how it can go awry, and the resulting difficulties and concerns experienced by their parents. It is only through this understanding that effective recommendations at a policy and individual level can emerge.

In this chapter I shall introduce the problem of failure to thrive, and discuss how the problem is so often poorly handled by health professionals. I shall attempt to explore why this is so, and describe the work of the Belmont House Growth and Nutrition Team in this area. In sharing my work and that of my colleagues, I hope that it will reach more parents and help them when facing difficulties in feeding their young children.

What Is Failure to Thrive?

Failure to thrive is a term used by health professionals to describe infants and young children who fail to gain weight adequately. The causes for poor weight gain are manifold, and, in general, the term failure to thrive relates to those children who have no underlying medical problem. As infant weight gain has always been seen as an indicator of a child's health and well-being, considerable anxiety is usually aroused when a baby "falls off centiles"[a] – and the principal concern is that irreversible damage may occur to the developing brain.

When young children fail to gain weight adequately, it is also very common to find that they have eating difficulties.[2] Parents often describe[3,4] that their children have poor appetites, are "picky" about what foods they will eat or have aversive reactions when being fed. (See quotes below.)

Parents' Descriptions of What It Was Like to Feed Their Child

- "I was winding (burping) him every ounce, and then the whole lot would come up and…I had to start all over again. You spend your whole day trying to get something inside him."
- "He wouldn't eat finger foods, he'd make himself sick, he had blended food for ages. It was just like a nightmare getting him to eat anything. He just wasn't interested."

[a]Babies' growth is monitored on growth charts, and usually tracks along a centile line. "Falling off a centile" implies that either weight or height gain is not satisfactory.

- "...She should be having at least a pint of milk a day, and I thought it was all I could do to get 4 ounces down her. I was in (an) absolute panic...."
- "...then after the meal, when you have had your big fight with them, you are narked (upset). 'Oh you spoilt little thing.' It takes...the full day...you are constantly trying to get them to eat."
- "It was more of a behavioural problem than a feeding problem. She wasn't eating a lot you know, she was getting down from the table and running around and playing.... Mealtimes were going on and on and on, and she wasn't putting on enough weight."

Given the already high levels of anxiety, the stress that develops around mealtimes is enormous. The imperative to encourage the child to eat any food is so high that the situation commonly deteriorates even further. Mealtimes often become stressful and drawn out. In fact, much of the day can be spent presenting food to the child, using bribery, games and even force feeding. (See parents' comment below.)

How Parents Feel When Their Child Has Eating Difficulties

- "...It feels hurtful. It feels like a rejection. (When) a mother gives her child, and the child doesn't want it, it (hurts)."
- "It was quite upsetting...me and my husband used to fall out over it. We had disagreements (and) we were both very concerned, but he took...more...action,...trying to force the food down him. It was devastating because we were rowing about how we were going to cope with him. Feeding time was a very stressful business."
- "It is just my whole life...it (feels) like it is you that is doing something wrong."
- "I felt more isolated than anything else. I mean I was a first-time mom as well, and you are stuck at home with this kid that doesn't eat anything."

The eating difficulties encountered in failure to thrive are not of course unique to failure to thrive, though they may be more extreme. Even when children are growing well, parents often perceive that their children are not eating enough. They fear that if their children do not eat regularly, they will not thrive. As a result, children are given the foods they like rather than those that comprise a healthy diet. Understanding parents' concerns and what happens around mealtime are therefore key to developing effective recommendations that are likely to have a positive impact on children's nutrition.

How Helpful Are Health Professionals When There Are Eating Problems?

Sadly there is plentiful evidence[3,4] that health professionals may not be helpful to parents as they manage their children's eating problems. (See quotes below.) If a child is growing well, health professionals are often dismissive. They provide parents with "reassurance" that all is well and that there is no need for concern, but leave them to struggle with mealtimes and their anxieties. When weight gain is poor, physicians and other health professionals have a tendency to be judgemental, conveying the attitude that failure to thrive is a result of poor parenting at best, and neglect or abuse at worst. The advice is often to simply offer more food, which may well aggravate the situation, especially when they give the message that brain growth and development will be jeopardised if the growth pattern does not improve.

Parents' Descriptions of the Help They Received From Healthcare Professionals Related to Their Children's Eating Problems

- "...it was a problem made worse by the healthcare professionals saying she's not eating enough, you have got to make her eat more.... After we saw the paediatrician, we became very concerned and we did everything to get food into her.... That's when she started to become even more stressed over food."

- "Both me and my husband felt we were to blame, we felt guilty, (and) they made (us) feel…as if we were somehow starving her, which we weren't. The paediatrician said there (was) nothing physically wrong so get more calories into her and that was that.…There was nothing else that they advised us. We went to the dietician, but she said to give her high calorie food, which we were trying to do anyway.…That was it.…There was no reason why she wasn't eating. We started to panic and it made her worse because we were trying to force feed her. She was very, very thin. We had to force feed her. It was scary."
- "I don't think the health visitor was that interested.…She said his weight was okay, so she wasn't that bothered. Although it was taking me a couple of hours to feed him…"
- "…They used to say, 'Well, put more in her bottle.' It was like I was the culprit…I wasn't giving her enough…"
- "I felt quite upset because they were accusing me of not feeding her…so I was going mad. Nobody took any notice of me."
- "…At one (point) I had the social worker coming, the health visitor coming and the doctor coming…and (I) was just lost…There was somebody there every day.…Everybody gave (me) different advice and then (I) didn't know whose to follow…"
- "When my daughter stopped putting on weight…she was weighed every week. It was over 18 months of them coming (to my home) and weighing her every week…and then saying, 'She will grow out of it.' After 18 months, she went 2 weeks without eating (anything) at all…I packed her bags up one day, took her down to the clinic, and said take her in hospital because I am not doing it anymore."

Why Do Health Professionals so Often Get It Wrong?

In order to gain an understanding of why health professionals may be unhelpful, it is instructive to take a historical perspective on our understanding of how infant growth relates to nutrition and the home environment.

The paediatric world began to appreciate that food alone is not adequate for good growth and well-being more than 100 years ago, when an American paediatrician, Henry Chapin, carried out a trial on babies and young children in institutions for the destitute.[5] At that time, the mortality rate among these infants and children was appalling — with as many as 50% of babies dying within their first year of life, despite being provided with adequate food. Chapin's research showed that these institutionalised children thrived when they were placed in foster care by the sea. This message was reinforced after World War II when Elsie Widdowson, a British nutritionist, conducted research in orphanages in Germany.[6] Widdowson wanted to see whether supplements of bread and jam could improve children's growth. To her surprise, she found that children who received the supplements of bread and jam did not grow as well as a control group of children who did not receive the supplements. The puzzle was solved when Widdowson discovered that the tyrant of a matron who ruled mealtimes in the control orphanage had been transferred to the intervention orphanage just as the supplements were introduced (see Figure 1). She concluded her beautifully written paper with a quote from Proverbs[7]:

"Better a dinner of herbs where love is than a fat ox with evil will."

Figure 1. The results of a trial conducted by Elsie Widdowson in German orphanages after World War II. After 6 months of following children's growth in the orphanages, bread supplements were given to the Vogelnest children. Surprisingly the control children in Bienenhaus grew better. She attributed this to the transfer of the tyrannical matron, Frau Schwartz, who moved from Bienenhaus to Vogelnest as supplementation was introduced.

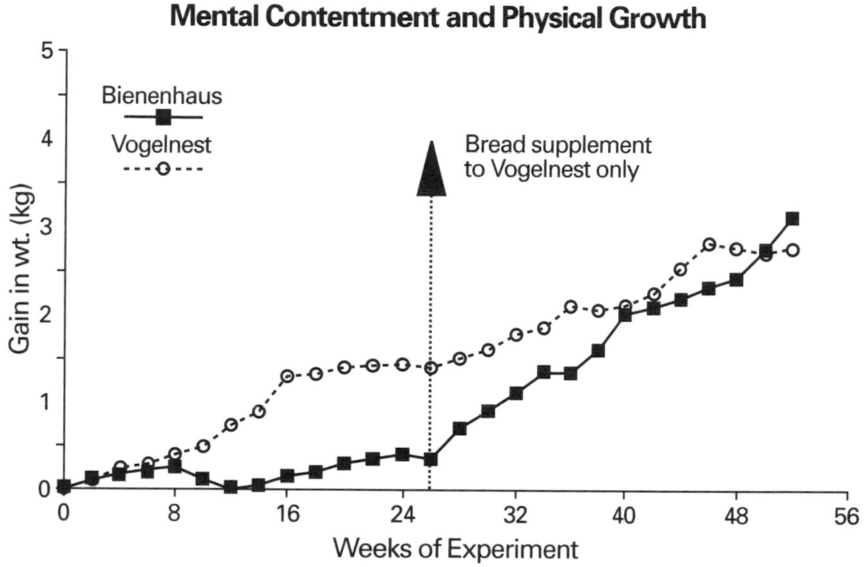

Reprinted from *The Lancet*, Vol 257, Widdowson EM, Mental contentment and physical growth, 1951, with permission from Elsevier.

By the 1970s, the emphasis that the home environment was critical for optimum growth and well-being turned towards a realisation that failure to thrive could be an important indicator of child abuse and neglect. Tragic cases such as that of Jasmine Beckford[8] (as illustrated in Figure 2), who died as a result of extreme neglect, despite the involvement of social services as a baby, strongly influenced health professionals and the approach they took when confronted by a child with poor growth. As a result, poor weight gain in an infant or young child is still commonly equated with poor parenting, and parents are often apportioned a combination of blame and responsibility for the lack of weight gain. To compound the situation, the message is likely to be

Figure 2. The growth chart of Jasmine Beckford, a little girl with failure to thrive who died as a result of neglect and abuse.

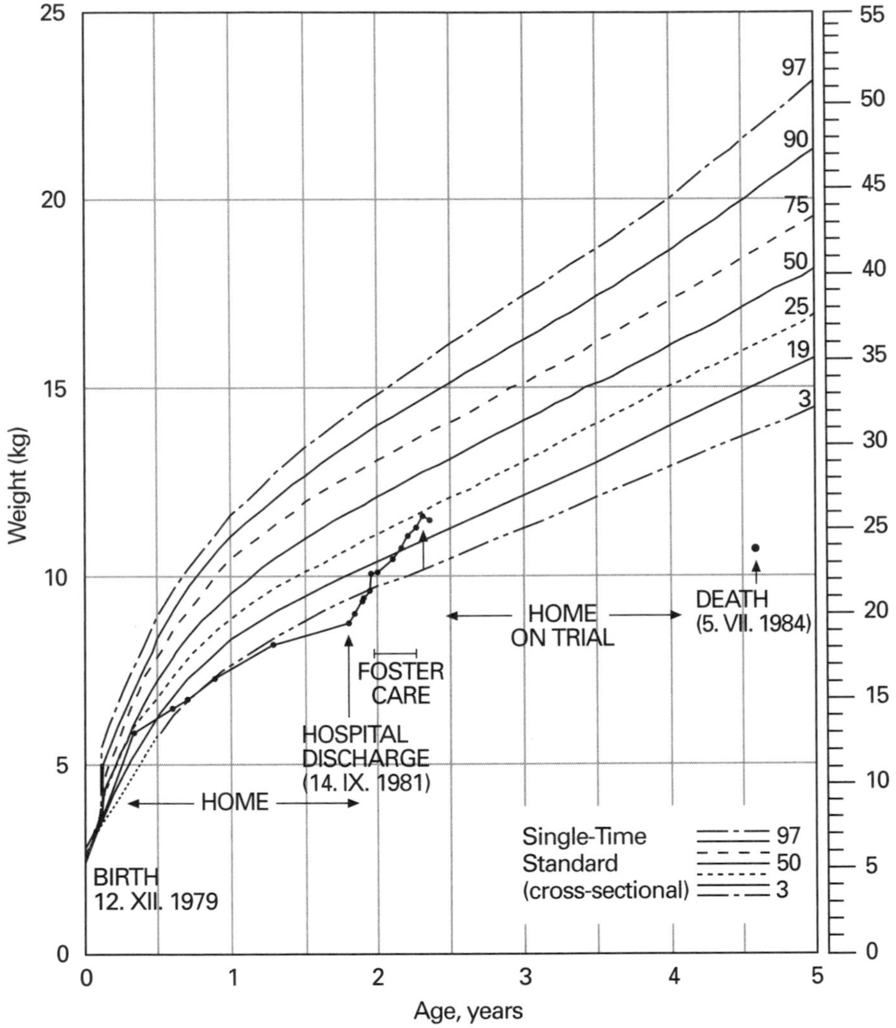

Reprinted from the Report of the Panel of Inquiry Into the Circumstances Surrounding the Death of Jasmine Beckford. Dec 1985. London HMSO.

conveyed to the parents that unless food intake is increased, brain damage will result. It is therefore not surprising that parents may find health professionals unhelpful and their own anxieties about their child's future exacerbated.

The Relationship Between Poor Weight Gain in Infancy and the Outcome in Childhood

Before looking into how health professionals might develop an approach that families would find helpful when dealing with concerns about their child's weight and eating difficulties, it is worthwhile to clarify what is known about the impact that poor weight gain has on a child's subsequent growth and development. A colleague and I conducted a systematic review of the literature[9] in an attempt to answer this question. We searched the literature for cohort studies of infants with poor weight gain who had been identified early, and followed through childhood, and were surprised to find that the outcomes were remarkably good. Although these children were somewhat shorter and thinner than comparison groups of normally growing infants, their growth was within the normal range, and, of key importance, their intellectual and behavioural outcomes were essentially comparable. (See Figure 3.)

Figure 3. Meta analysis of intellectual scores in children who had experienced failure to thrive in infancy compared with controls.

	Failure to thrive		Controls		SMD*	Weight	WMD*
Study	n	mean (sd)	n	mean (sd)	(95% CI)	%	(95% CI)
Boddy 2000	42	99.8 (15.9)	42	103.7 (19.7)		19.6	-0.22 [-0.65,0.21]
Corbett 1996	48	83.6 (11.5)	46	87.0 (11.9)		21.8	-0.29 [-0.07,0.12]
Drewett 1999	107	87.6 (17.4)	117	90.6 (17.1)		52.3	-0.17 (-0.44,0.09)
Mitchell 1980	12	87.5 (12.9)	16	92.5 (12.9		6.3	-0.38 (-1.13,0.38)
Total (95% CI)	209		221			100.0	-0.22 [-0.41,-0.03]

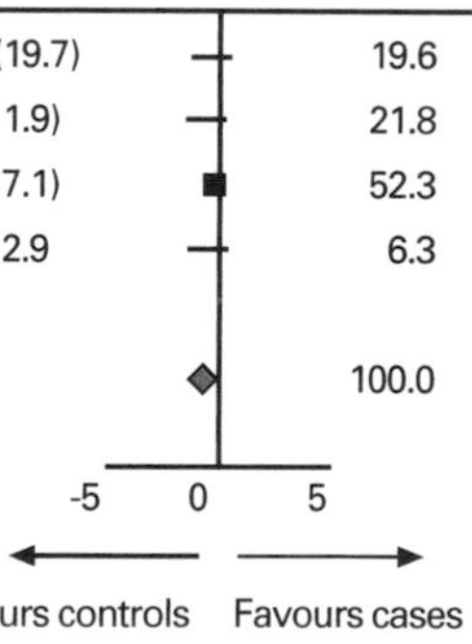

*SMD standardised mean difference WMD weighted mean difference

The message to be drawn from this systematic literature review is that the outcome for the majority of children with weight faltering[b] is good, and that the anxiety generated by health professionals is often excessive and certainly unhelpful. This does not mean that poor growth, particularly when extreme, should not be a concern. It may well be a marker for conditions where growth and developmental outcomes are poor. However, our research suggests that the assumption that poor weight gain in infancy inevitably leads to subsequent problems is flawed.

So, if poor weight gain does not necessarily affect a child's potential, can we assume that nutrition is unimportant in infancy? This would clearly be inappropriate. Evidence is increasingly emerging that the nutrition given to infants is critical for subsequent health and well being.[10] There is also the concern that the poor quality diets that babies receive at weaning is contributing heavily to the epidemic of obesity that we are facing today. However, the message that we need to take from our systematic review is that brain damage is not a necessary consequence of poor weight gain, and that it is unhelpful for professionals to underpin their advice to parents with this message.

The Belmont House Growth and Nutrition Team

The Belmont House Growth and Nutrition Team was established in Leeds, England, in 1993 to provide a clinical service to families with babies and children who were failing to thrive. In the mid-1990s the team received funding to conduct a trial to determine whether intensive home visiting could improve the outcome of these children.[2] The results of this research have profoundly shaped our practice and our approach to the families that are referred to our service.

Over the course of the trial we found that parents who were visited at home greatly appreciated the support and advice provided by the specialist health visitor. Analysis of a questionnaire on children's eating habits completed by parents at baseline and again after the home visits showed a significant reduction in the severity of children's eating problems, an improvement in appetites and that mealtimes were more relaxed (Figure 4).[11] However, it is noteworthy that our primary outcomes of growth and development were no different from children who had received standard outpatient care.[11]

[b]Some professionals feel that the term "weight faltering" should replace "failure to thrive," as they consider the latter is pejorative, and may imply that parents are failing in their role.

Figure 4. A reduction in eating difficulties in 83 children with failure to thrive.[11]

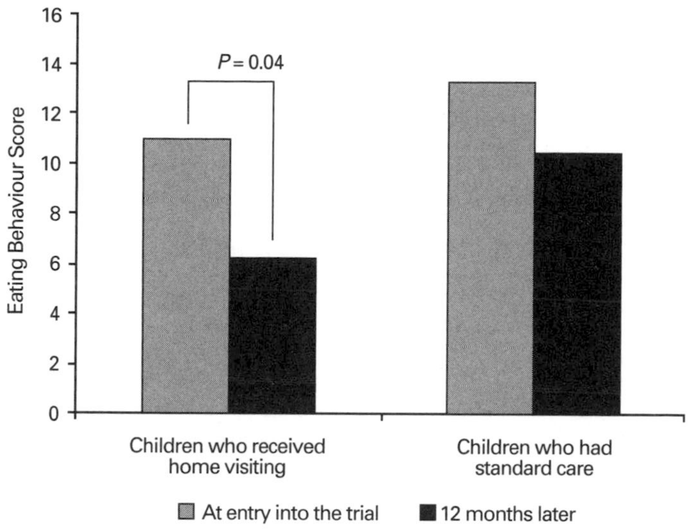

Working With Parents and Children

The Growth and Nutrition Team centres around a specialist health visitor, whose key input relies on an in-depth assessment of the issues concerning the parents, carers and other health professionals. The assessment is carried out in the child's home and includes observation of a mealtime by the specialist health visitor. In addition, each child under the care of the team undergoes a paediatric assessment to ensure that there is no medical cause for their poor growth and eating difficulties. When appropriate, the family and child are referred to a psychologist, dietician and dentist.

Two tools that my colleagues and I developed — the mealtime video and the personal questionnaire — shed light on how young children eat and what may go wrong, and also on the sort of concerns and issues that parents commonly face. In addition to these insights, these tools also offer a way to reach out to parents in this emotive area. Although the tools were developed for use with children who are failing to thrive, we have no doubt that they are also relevant to understanding and helping any family confronted with young children's eating difficulties, whether of a behavioural nature or where under-nutrition or overeating is a concern.

The Mealtime Video

The experience gained in videoing mealtimes for research purposes brought us to the realisation that we had much to learn about the issues confronting families. An assessment in a paediatric clinic — which had been the standard for understanding children's eating behaviours — could not begin to uncover the sort of difficulties that parents and children were experiencing. These videos proved to be of value not only to the health visitor assessing the child, but to the mother herself. As a result the team has adopted the practice of having both the health visitor and the mother view the video together after the meal. In doing so, the mother can see how her interaction with her child may be exacerbating the situation rather than encouraging the child to eat better. She can then begin to appreciate the cues that the child is giving related to eating, gain a better understanding of what may help her child and begin to adjust mealtimes so they become less stressful for the entire family. The result is usually that the child begins to eat better.

We began to realise that the mealtime video is a potentially powerful educational tool for health professionals too. With the willing agreement of mothers, we developed a teaching package for health professionals[c] based on some of the audiovisual vignettes accompanied by background information on the child and the family. The health professionals viewing the tapes are encouraged to systematically analyse the vignettes by focusing on the child, the parent, the interaction between the two, the setting of the meal and the nutritional quality of the food. By so doing they develop an understanding of the issues that may contribute to eating difficulties as well as formulate a coherent approach to tackling them.

[c]The audiovisual pack *Clues From Children's Mealtimes: Insights Into Managing Infant and Toddler Eating Behaviour* is available from Media Services, University of Leeds, Leeds LS2 9JT.
Tel: +44 (0)113 343 2660, Fax +44 (0)113 343 2669.

When health professionals are shown the vignettes, they are often taken aback by what they see. The vignettes provide them with eyewitness accounts of eating difficulties that are hard to grasp in a brief clinical encounter. By appreciating and taking into account what actually happens at children's mealtimes, health professionals can help parents take the necessary steps to improve their children's eating behaviour and nutrition.

The Personal Questionnaire

Because standard psychological measures did not adequately address and capture families' concerns regarding eating difficulties, my colleagues and I explored other methods that might suit our purpose better. We have found that using personal questionnaires[12] are of value both as a research and clinical tool. They have offered us insights into the stresses and tensions that occur within a family when a child eats poorly, and how this environment may result in unbalanced, unhealthy diets.

Personal questionnaires are a simple concept. They are individualised questionnaires that are compiled by the clinician in partnership with the children's parent(s) or carer. Together, the clinician and parent itemise the parent or carer's concerns about the child and the impact that the child's eating difficulties have on the family. Once the questionnaire has been compiled and agreed upon, the parent scores the concerns for their severity. Periodically the parent is then asked to rescore the concerns on the questionnaire (without seeing earlier scores at the time), and add new concerns if they arise. Over time, a pattern emerges as to whether these issues are being resolved or intensifying. An example of a personal questionnaire is shown in Figure 5, with a demonstration as to how it changed over the course of several months.

Figure 5. Parents' Concerns Summary Sheet.

Belmont House Growth and Nutrition Team
Personal Questionnaire - Summary Sheet

Parent's Name: ______________________
Child's Name: ______________________
Date of Birth: ______________________
Name of Scorer: ______________________

Scoring:
4 = Very Considerable, 3 = Moderate to Considerable, 2 = Slight to Considerable, 1 = Very Slight

Date of Visit		07 08 01	03 10 01	14 02 02	29 04 02	02 07 02	24 09 02	02 12 02	21 01 03	05 03 03	
1	The feeling that mealtimes are stressful	4	3	3	3	2	2	3	2	1	
2	Concern that what Adam eats causes arguments between myself and my husband	3	2	2	2	1	1	1	2	1	
3	Concern about something being wrong medically with Adam's throat or stomach	4	3	4	3	2	1	2	2	1	
4	The feeling that it is something I have done	3	3	2	2	2	1	3	2	1	
5	A tendency to force feed Adam which makes me feel bad	4	2	3	2	3	1	2	2	1	
6	The feeling that mealtimes are desperate	4	3	3	2	3	1	4	2	1	
7	Concern about distracting Adam with toys and playing in the garden to get him to eat	3	2	3	2	3	1	2	2	1	
8	The feeling that life revolves around Adam	4	2	3	3	3	1	4	3	1	
9	The feeling that I can't go anywhere	4	2	3	3	2	1	3	2	1	
10	Concern about what Adam will be like when he starts school	4	3	4	3	3	2	3	2	1	
11	Concern about whether Adam will ever be able to feed himself	4	3	3	3	3	1	4	2	1	
12	Concern that Adam is in control	4	4	4	4	3	2	4	3	1	
13	Concern about Adam's behaviour	4	4	4	3	3	2	3	3	2	

Additional Notes

In 2004 we reviewed the personal questionnaires of 34 parents who received home visiting.[13] Our findings are shown in Table 1. The concerns we had elicited in the questionnaires emphasise the impact a child's eating difficulties has on the entire family. When professional input into failure to thrive focuses on nutritional advice alone, one can see why parents find this unhelpful. Gratifyingly, following a period of home visiting, the majority of parents showed a decrease in the intensity of their concerns.

Table 1. Concerns documented by parents of children with failure to thrive in compiling their personal questionnaires. A score of 3 or 4 indicates concerns at a "clinical level." After a period of home visiting, the number of parents with these high scores decreased.

Category of concern	Concern	No. of carers with scores of 3 or 4 at initial visit	No. of carers with scores of 3 or 4 at last visit
Feeding and mealtimes	The type of food eaten	20	10
	Mealtimes are stressful	13	3
	The amount of food eaten	12	7
Explanations of what's the matter	The child not gaining weight/FTT	10	6
	The possibility of a medical problem	5	0
	Perception that the child is in control	3	4
Impact on family life	Arguments between partners	18	1
	Life revolving around feeding	7	5
	Effect on other children in the family	5	2
	Embarrassment about the feeding problem	3	0
Solutions and stuckness	The use of distraction or bribery to get the child to eat	7	2
	Force feeding	3	0
Me and my life	Negative effects on parents	15	1
Fears about the future	General concerns about the future	13	9
	Concern about starting school	3	1
	Concern about future health and development	1	0
The situation in general	The feeling of being under pressure about feeding	9	3
Professionals and people's help	Negative comments about professionals	6	2

One of the advantages of using personal questionnaires is that progress becomes evident to both the parent and the clinician, and any unresolved concerns that continue to be troublesome can be revisited. This process allows the intervention to focus on the family's issues rather than the clinician's agenda. The value of personal questionnaires was confirmed when we surveyed the parents of our patients through anonymised postal questionnaires. Their responses strongly affirmed that the process was helpful. Parents felt that through the process of jointly compiling the personal questionnaire with a health visitor, they felt listened to and they themselves became clearer about their concerns. They reported that the personal questionnaire made sure that there was focus on these concerns at each visit, that the concerns were addressed, and that it helped to see how they progressed over time.

Videotapes of mealtimes and the results from the personal questionnaires offer some insight into what really happens around young children's mealtimes, the issues families face and the depth of concern and anxiety that parents face. Given that as many as 1 in 6 very young children have significant eating difficulties,[14] these issues are likely to be very widespread. The sort of advice that we offer to parents of our patients is shown below.

Advice Given to Parents Attending the Belmont House Growth and Nutrition Service When There Are Concerns About Poor Weight Gain

Managing Mealtimes

- Help your child to become more involved in the feeding process by encouraging touching and playing with food, even if it is very messy.
- Try to provide a relaxed, calm atmosphere at mealtimes.
- Encourage the family to eat together as children learn by example.
- If your child shows interest in what others are eating, allow him or her to share it.
- Limit mealtimes to 30 minutes and remove food without comment. Longer mealtimes rarely result in more food being eaten.

- Ignore bad behaviour at mealtimes by turning away from the child.
- Praise the child for eating.

Nutrition and Diet

- Start with food that is familiar to the child even if interest is only shown in a limited variety of foods.
- Offer a small portion of food to start with and if readily eaten, offer more. Some children have a small appetite.
- Offering meals and snacks frequently will help to stimulate the appetite.
- Offer high-calorie foods, which are important for growth in young children. (eg, use full-fat milk, cheese, yogurt and butter. These can be added to mashed potato, pasta, etc.)
- Make sure your child has only 20 oz of milk per day once he/she is over 12 months of age, and only 2 cups of juice. Some children fill up on drinks throughout the day.
- Limit daytime use of a pacifier because it can affect food intake and language development.
- If your child is slow at eating, gently encourage but never force feed.

Applying the Belmont House Approach to Overweight Children

The work of the Belmont House Growth and Nutrition Team described in this chapter was developed for children who eat poorly, and where under-nutrition is the chief concern. Might this be of any relevance to the epidemic of obesity that we are now facing? Now that parents and health professionals are becoming aware that rapid weight gain in infancy is associated with childhood obesity, we are receiving referrals for obese infants and toddlers. We are finding that the issues are not dissimilar from those faced by parents with children who fail to thrive:

- As with poor weight gain, the family circumstances are generally complex.
- Many of the infants have large appetites that seem to be insatiable and parental attempts to limit food intake are greeted with crying that can try the best of parenting skills.
- Other infants are overfed as a result of parents failing to interpret their infants' cues.
- Some have a narrow range of food preferences, so that attempts to provide a healthier diet are beset with difficulty.
- Families may be confronted by health professionals who apportion blame to the parents.[15,16]

We are currently piloting the use of videos at mealtimes with obese infants and are beginning to learn more about the eating behaviour and mealtime interaction that occur at this end of the feeding and nutrition spectrum. Like failure to thrive, reading infants' cues is critical. Personal questionnaires provide a further opportunity for understanding families' issues, which may differ in some respects but will no doubt emphasise the tensions and anxieties that may arise when a child begins to gain excessive weight.

Discussion

Today, because messages regarding the importance of a healthy balanced diet are being widely broadcasted, lack of nutritional knowledge is rarely the principal barrier. Most parents are fully aware of what their children should eat, the problem is how to encourage them to do so. The central issue is one of parenting.

The challenge for those with expertise in child feeding and nutrition is to develop practical recommendations for parents, health professionals and policymakers. To do so, we need to recognise the difficulties and concerns of parents around their children's eating. By incorporating their perspective, we may hope to develop effective recommendations that parents will follow to optimise children's diets. This has gained increasing importance now that we are aware how obesity and its attendant eating behaviours may have their onset in the early years.

Scevole de Ste Marthe described over 400 years ago how eating difficulties can arise and challenge parents, causing despair when their child fails to eat according to plan. Tackling children's eating behaviours through enhancing parenting will have a profound impact not only on the nutritional state of children but on family well-being too.

Acknowledgments

I would like to acknowledge my colleagues in the Growth and Nutrition Team at Belmont House in Leeds. Dr Pauline Raynor, specialist health visitor, conducted the randomised controlled trial of home visiting for failure to thrive for her doctoral thesis, and extended this work to ascertain parents' views and developed *Clues From Children's Mealtimes.* Bernadette Mulley, specialist health visitor, developed the use of personal questionnaires, under the encouragement and guidance of Jack Chalkley, clinical psychologist in Avon and Wiltshire NHS Trust. Dr Terence Gaussen, clinical psychologist, Dr Fauzia Khan and Dr Karen Naylor, community paediatricians, and Zofia Smith, paediatric dietitian, all contributed energy into supporting this research while running a busy clinical service. Thanks also to Professor Sir David Hall who, over the years, has given us such encouragement in our work.

References

1. De Ste Marthe SG. *Paedotrophia.* Tytler HW, trans-ed. London, England; 1795.
2. Raynor P, Rudolf MCJ, Cooper K, Marchant P, Cottrell D. A randomized controlled trial of specialist health visitor intervention for failure to thrive. *Archives of Disease in Childhood.* 1999;80:500-506.
3. Raynor P. *Failure to Thrive: Are Outcomes Improved by a Specialist Health Visitor - A Randomized Controlled Trial* [doctoral thesis]. Leeds, England: University of Leeds; 2002.
4. Underdown A. *When Feeding Fails: Parents' Experiences of Faltering Growth.* London, England: The Children's Society; 2000.
5. Chapin HD. Are institutions for infants necessary? *Journal of the American Medical Association.* 1908;64:1-3.
6. Widdowson E. Mental contentment and physical growth. *Lancet.* 1951;1:1316-1318.
7. Proverbs 15:17.
8. Beal J, Blom-Cooper L, Brown B, Marshall P, Mason M. *A Child in Trust. The Report of the Panel of Inquiry Into the Circumstances Surrounding the Death of Jasmine Beckford.* Middlesex, England: Kingswood Press; 1985.
9. Rudolf MCJ, Logan S. What is the long-term outcome for children who fail to thrive? A systematic review. *Archives of Disease in Childhood.* 2005;90:925-931.
10. Lucas A. Long-term programming effects of early nutrition — implications for the preterm infant. *Journal of Perinatology.* 2005;suppl 2:S2-S6.
11. Raynor P, Rudolf MCJ, Cottrell D, Cooper K, Marchant P. An RCT of focused intervention and its effect on mealtime and eating behaviour in families with children diagnosed as failing to thrive. *Archives of Disease in Childhood.* 1999;80:suppl 1:A62.
12. Chalkley AJ. The description of concerns. *Psychology and Psychotherapy: Theory, Research and Practice.* 2004;77:207-230.
13. Mulley B, Rudolf MCJ, Chalkley J. "Personal Questionnaires — A Better Way to Listen to the Concerns of Parents Whose Child Is Failing to Thrive": Report for BUPA (British United Provident Association), 2003. Obtainable from author, Community Paediatrics, Belmont House, 3-5 Belmont Grove, Leeds, LS2 9DE, England.
14. Polnay L, Hull D. *Community Pediatrics.* London, England: Churchill Livingstone; 1993.
15. Dixey R, Rudolf MCJ, Murtagh J. WATCH IT obesity management for children: a qualitative exploration of the views of parents. *Archives of Disease in Childhood* [serial online]. July 4, 2006.
16. Edmunds LD. Parents' perceptions of health professionals' responses when seeking help for their overweight children. *Family Practice.* 2005;22:287-292.

Using Childcare Programs as a Portal for Changing the Eating Behaviors of Young Children

Richard Fiene, PhD

Introduction

Given the epidemic of overweight and obesity among children, helping them to eat better is an important goal. There are few interventions that are effective in dealing with childhood overweight and obesity. This chapter outlines an intervention that has proven to be effective based on randomized clinical trials.

Why use childcare as an entry point for dealing with the issue of overweight and obesity among children? Because today the majority of preschool-age children participate in some form of childcare — and eat 1 or more of their daily meals during that time. Five years ago, we began to see this demographic shift. Therefore, childcare programs are a natural portal for interventions targeted to young children and their families.

Many types of interventions related to childcare and childhood obesity have already been instituted at the state, regional and local levels. Several state and regional approaches are discussed briefly in the next section of this chapter. These are very broad-based public policy initiatives that lack empirical support for their effectiveness. At the local level, workshops, classes, seminars, technical assistance and, most recently, mentoring sessions seek to address childhood obesity. For the most part, their effectiveness has also not been tested. This chapter focuses specifically on mentoring because it has been demonstrated to be the most effective in producing behavioral change in childcare settings.

The Effectiveness of Mentoring: A Randomized Clinical Trial of Mentoring in Childcare

The use of mentoring in childcare has been documented in the literature for the past 10 to 15 years.[1,2] It has been demonstrated to be an effective mode of training.[1] Many studies on mentoring track the progress of the intervention; some studies included comparison groups, but few, if any, employed a truly randomized clinical trial design. This chapter describes the pre- and posttest data collected as part of a randomized clinical trial on mentoring in childcare[3] and suggests how content relevant to children's eating behaviors could be introduced into the model.

This study in south central Pennsylvania[3] — to demonstrate the effectiveness of a mentoring approach with infant/toddler caregivers — involved 40 caregivers from 20 childcare sites licensed by the Pennsylvania Department of Public Welfare (Southcentral Pennsylvania Infant Child Care Provider Mentoring Study, supported by the Pennsylvania Department of Public Welfare, July 2000–June 2003). The results reported in this chapter are from the pre- and posttest data-collection phase of the study, and include descriptive data on individual programs, program directors and caregivers, as well as comparisons among programs.

Childcare Program Statistics

The average age of the directors of childcare programs participating in this study was 33 years of age, with a range from 24 to 51 years of age. The directors were predominantly white (80%). Their level of education varied: 8% reported to have an associate degree, 60% a bachelor's degree and 32% a master's degree. The directors had been employed by their programs for an average of 29 months, with a range from 5 to 130 months. Overall, although the directors were fairly young, they had a significant amount of on-the-job experience and were well-educated individuals.

Other descriptive statistics on the program directors include the following:

- Salaries ranged from $22,000 to $27,000 per year

- Some 62% were provided health insurance and 57% were provided some form of dental or life insurance
- Some 65% were provided a retirement plan

The average age of the caregivers in the childcare programs participating in this study was 35 years of age, with a range of 20 to 64 years of age. The caregivers were predominantly white (70%). Some 47% of the caregivers reported having a high school diploma, 26% some college credit, 13% an associate degree, 8% a bachelor's degree, 5% a Child Development Associate certificate and 2% a master's degree. The caregivers had been employed by their programs for an average of 37 months, with a range of 4 to 144 months. They had worked in the early childhood field for 75 months on average, with a range of 4 to 220 months.

Other descriptive statistics on the caregivers include the following:

- Annual pay ranged from $12,000 to $17,500
- Some 55% were provided health insurance and 43% were provided some form of dental or life insurance
- Some 43% were provided a retirement plan

The average size of the childcare programs participating in the study was 95 children and 17 staff employed on either a full-time or part-time basis. The average weekly fee was $157 for infant care and $134 for toddler care.

Study Design

The study employed a truly randomized design: 20 participating childcare programs were randomly assigned to 1 of 2 groups, either the mentoring group or a control group without mentoring. From September to December 2001, staff in the mentoring group received intensive mentoring from a seasoned early childhood professional. That individual had many years of experience in the early childhood field as both a childcare program director and a teacher. The control group received routine in-service training, which included workshop training that was available in the local community, but they did not receive the mentoring intervention. However, the control group did subsequently receive the mentoring intervention from March to June

2002. The study sought to determine how the 2 groups changed from the pretest data-collection period (September 2001 to June 2002) — when they were essentially equivalent — to after the mentoring period.

To assess changes in the caregivers, the study used 4 data-collection and measurement tools:

- Infant Toddler Environmental Rating Scale (ITERS), a global measure of infant classroom quality
- Arnett Caregiver Observation Scale, a measure that rates the interactions between children and their caregivers
- Knowledge of Infant Development Inventory (KIDI), a measure that gives an indication of the overall knowledge that an individual has of infant development
- Bloom Program Administration Scale, a measure that rates the overall organizational climate of a childcare center

Study Results

The similarity of the mentoring and control groups was assessed during the pretest data-collection phase. During this phase, the 2 groups showed no statistically significant differences on any of the 4 measures. When the programs and caregivers were measured again at posttest, the results were significantly different. In the aggregate, the programs that continued with the mentoring project (n = 20) showed improvements in the overall quality of care. There was a +0.50 increase on the ITERS; a +0.35 increase on the Arnett; a 10% increase on the KIDI; and a 7-point increase on the Bloom scale. Four caregivers (10%) dropped out of the project between pre- and posttest: 2 in the mentoring group and 2 in the control group. The programs that received the mentoring intervention had as much difficulty retaining staff as did the control-group programs. The only factor that correlated highly with staff retention was the salary of the caregiver (r = .68). There was a strong relationship between staff salaries and the ITERS score (.77) and Arnett (.45) score: The higher the salaries, the higher the rating of overall program quality and child/caregiver interactions.

When the data are broken out by mentoring versus comparison group, a very different picture emerges. (See Table 1.)

Table 1. Results on 4 Measures for the Mentoring Intervention Group (n = 18) and Control Group (n = 22)

	Pretest		Posttest		Change	
Measure	**Intervention**	**Control**	**Intervention**	**Control**	**Intervention**	**Control**
ITERS	3.89	4.05	4.74	4.00	+0.85*	(-0.05)
Arnett	3.33	3.36	3.84	3.50	+.51	+.14
KIDI	70%	70%	90%	70%	+20%*	-0-
Bloom	83	87	94	91	+11	+4.0

$^{*}P<.01$

These results, which are statistically significant ($P<.01$), are important because the mentoring group showed strong positive increases on the 4 measures, while the control group remained the same, showed a small decrease or increased slightly. In the control group sites, the measure of overall global quality (ITERS) dropped from a score of 4.05 to 4.00. On the Arnett scale, the mentoring group increased more than the control group did (ie, a .51-point increase in the intervention group versus a .14-point increase in the control group). Although the results for the overall measures did not reach statistical significance in all cases, when the data were broken out by individual items measured by each tool, many of these did reach statistical significance. (See Tables 2 and 3.)

It appears that mentoring had a positive effect for all of the intervention programs, but it worked best in those programs in which the staff was most receptive (the teacher and director thought the mentoring would be helpful, rather than just the director thinking the mentoring would be helpful). When the programs were grouped by overall quality (eg, a high group with high quality and a low group with lower quality), the high group improved significantly more than did the low group. In some cases, the high group increased by 2.50 points on the ITERS. Although the low group showed improvement, there were more obstacles to overcome and thus the gains were

Table 2. Results for the Intervention Group for Items Contained Within 2 Measurement Tools

Tool and Areas Measured	Pretest	Posttest	Significance
ITERS:			
Routines	4.03	5.21	.005
Listening activities	3.77	4.50	.05
Learning activities	4.00	4.71	.05
Interactions	3.89	4.91	.01
Adult needs	4.10	4.70	.05
Arnett:			
Sensitivity	3.33	3.90	.001
Appropriate discipline	3.40	3.70	.05

Table 3. Results for the Control Group for Items Contained Within 2 Measurement Tools

Tool and Areas Measured	Pretest	Posttest	Significance
ITERS:			
Routines	4.10	4.20	—
Listening activities	4.01	3.89	—
Learning activities	3.99	4.11	—
Interactions	4.00	3.56	.02
Adult needs	3.90	3.90	—
Arnett:			
Sensitivity	3.46	3.50	—
Appropriate discipline	3.33	3.34	—

less than in the high group. In the low group, the teachers were not as motivated to make the changes suggested by the mentors because from the beginning they were volunteered by their director rather than this being a mutual decision by the director and teacher.

The data clearly demonstrate that the sites that were mentored improved significantly on the ITERS and Arnett measures. This is particularly important given that the intervention was only 4 to 5 months long and the individuals in the mentored group had lower scores on the Bloom scale preintervention. Another interesting result was the relationship between the Bloom scale and the ITERS and the Arnett scales. There were significant relationships between the Bloom scale (measures of professional development) and the ITERS (n = .56; $P<.01$) and Arnett (n = .46; $P<.01$) scales.

The overall organizational climate of the center appears to have an influence on how a program's quality increases over time. More than 40% of the variance in overall quality of childcare programs was accounted for by how staff felt decisions were made at the center (eg, whether they had self-sufficiency in making decisions) and how closely the center came to the ideal for staff pay and promotion opportunities, relationships with co-workers, agreement among staff on program goals, innovativeness and creative problem solving.

These data clearly demonstrate how the mentored programs improved from the pretest to the posttest on several program quality measures. This is an important finding because historically the majority of mentoring projects have relied on anecdotal evidence to demonstrate their effectiveness. Very few programs have conducted randomized trials of their mentoring interventions.

The data indicate that training and technical assistance interventions are needed in infant/toddler programs because of the low scores these programs received on various program quality measures. Without interventions, the quality of these programs may actually worsen over time. This is a hypothesis that is supported by data from other studies.[4]

An interesting finding was the strong relationship between organizational climate scores on the Bloom scale and the overall program quality scales — the ITERS and the Arnett. Previous research has shown the importance of commitment to professional development and the overall quality of the childcare program.[4] Data from this study support this initial finding. The findings in this study build upon the findings of previous studies[5] and demonstrate the importance of an organizational climate that supports openness and self-sufficiency in decision making.

Public Policy Implications

The public policy implications of the findings from this randomized clinical trial are significant because they demonstrate that a mentoring intervention can produce positive changes in the quality of childcare programs. Previous research[5] has indicated that interventions that increase the number of hours of training provided to staff result in staff interactions with children that are consistently more developmentally appropriate. Mentoring fits within this model because it is an intensive one-on-one intervention in which the mentor and the individual who is mentored are engaged in problem-solving activities to improve the quality of the staff-child interactions and the overall environment of the childcare program.

An additional public policy implication is that even when the best training (eg, intensive mentoring) is provided to childcare staff, it is unlikely to positively affect turnover in the long run. The results of this study suggest that the only factor that impacts turnover is the salary of the staff: The higher the salary of staff, the lower the turnover rate. In addition, greater than 56% of the variance in overall program quality is accounted for by staff salaries. Therefore, the issue of staff compensation in the childcare setting must be addressed. If it is not, well-trained staff will continue to leave their employment, and children will not reap the benefits of care-provider training.

In summary, from a public policy perspective, this research study indicates that the most important factors for improving the overall quality of childcare programs include the following:

- Training that is targeted through a mentoring approach (70 to 85 hours at a minimum over 4 months)
- An educated program director (with at least a bachelor's degree in early childhood education and state teaching certification)
- Experienced caregivers (with 5 years or more in the childcare field)
- Appropriate compensation (eg, $20,000 to $25,000 annually for caregivers/teachers and $30,000 to $35,000 for directors)
- A program director who has an open-minded decision-making process in which she or he is willing to engage teaching staff in all decisions related to professional development

Statewide Study of Childcare Quality and Nutrition-Related Activities

In a statewide study of early childcare and education[6] that obtained global assessments of quality, my colleagues and I found a disturbing result. In more than 70% of childcare centers where nutrition-related activities were measured, the following occurred:

- The meal/snack schedule was inappropriate (eg, a child is made to wait to eat, even if hungry)
- Food served was of unacceptable nutritional value
- Sanitary conditions were not usually maintained (eg, most children and/or adults did not wash hands before handling food, tables were not sanitized, toileting/diapering and food preparation areas were not separated)
- There was a negative social atmosphere around eating (eg, staff enforced manners harshly, children were forced to eat)
- No accommodations were made for children's food allergies

These are important and distressing findings. In the programs where these situations occurred, none had a mentoring program in place when these results were collected.

Similar results were found for in-home childcare as well. In this same study, the following situations were present in 85% of in-home childcare programs:

- Meal/snack schedule was irregular
- Cooking and eating areas were not kept clean
- Infants were not held for feedings and were routinely fed by propping a bottle
- Infants and toddlers were put to bed with bottles
- The nutritional quality of food was questionable

These childcare programs, both at centers and in homes, could benefit from a mentoring program, which was not available to them when this study was performed. A key benefit of mentoring is that it can be very flexible with content of the program. Mentoring can easily include specific components that deal with children's eating. In fact, nutritional modules have been built into both center-based and in-home mentoring programs. If this type of mentoring intervention were available to the programs in the study just described, the results could have been very different. The next section of this chapter discusses nutrition content in mentoring, as well as specific mentoring modules.

A series of studies conducted by Fiene[3] demonstrated that traditional workshop training for caregivers is not effective. When workshop instruction is linked with certificate programs that require a minimum of 24 hours of instruction, the certificate programs are more effective in producing behavioral change in caregivers. However, the most significant and longest-lasting behavioral changes in caregivers were found when these caregivers participated in mentoring programs of various lengths. The programs that were most effective in producing positive, developmentally appropriate changes in young children (based on the Developmental Observation Checklist System, or DOCS[7]) involved mentoring of the child's caregiver, their parents and the childcare director. Figure 1 demonstrates this relationship. (DOCS is a comprehensive developmental assessment of young children from infancy to preschool. The purpose of the DOCS is to identify infants and children who are developing normally and those significantly below their peers in acquiring cognitive, language, social and motor abilities; to give direction to instructional practice; and to document educational progress.)

Figure 1. DOCS scores of children based on caregiver training.

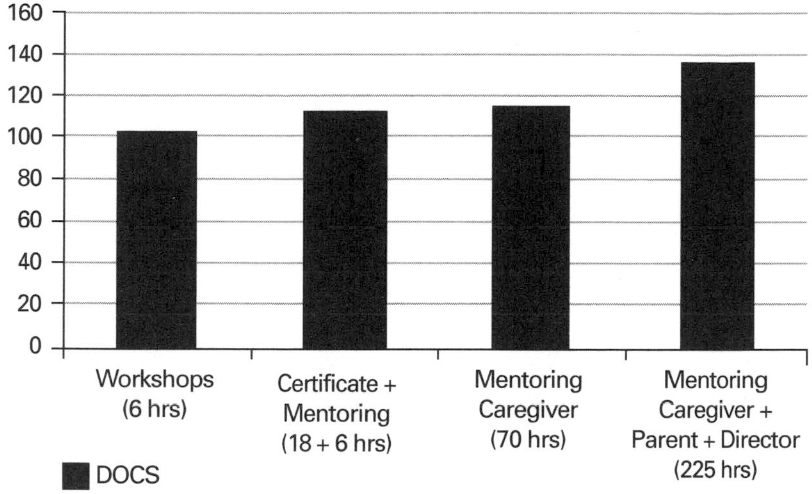

States' Initiatives Related to Childhood Obesity

At a state level, there are a number of public policy initiatives that deal with childhood obesity. North Carolina, New York and Texas have implemented innovative efforts to deal with this issue at a more global level than the mentoring intervention described above.

North Carolina

Color Me Healthy[8] is a joint effort of the North Carolina Cooperative Extension Service and the North Carolina Governor's Council on Physical Fitness and Health. These 2 lead organizations also partnered with the Start with Your Heart program and the North Carolina Initiative for Healthy Weight in Children and Adolescents. Start with Your Heart program is a statewide task force to reduce the incidence of heart attacks and strokes in North Carolina. The North Carolina Initiative for Healthy Weight in Children and Adolescents is a statewide initiative to address the problem of childhood obesity in North Carolina. County extension agents are asked to bring a partner of their choice to training in December. Family and Consumer Science agents, who are state employees, in the past, have partnered with local health departments, childcare resource and referral agencies, Healthy Carolinians (Healthy Carolinians is an effort to develop community-based partnerships to improve health in North Carolina; established in 1994, Healthy Carolinians is based on community engagement principles), local Fitness Councils or community volunteers. *Color Me Healthy* is designed to reach children 4 to 5 years of age with fun and interactive learning opportunities. It provides caregivers in childcare programs with quick and easy tools to teach young children about healthy eating and physical activity.

New York

Eat Well Play Hard,[9] an initiative spearheaded by the New York Department of Health, seeks to prevent overweight and the accompanying long-term risks of chronic disease, such as diabetes and coronary heart disease, by modifying behavior in preschoolers beginning at 2 years of age. The Department of Health provides funds to childcare programs and public schools to ensure that preschool and early elementary-age children and their families receive consistent and positive messages about nutrition and physical activity. Families are encouraged to adopt the following strategies to achieve life-long healthy choices:

- Increase the amount of developmentally appropriate physical activity
- Increase consumption of 1% or nonfat milk and low-fat dairy products
- Increase consumption of fruits and vegetables

Texas

The *Building Healthy Families Initiative*[10] was launched in September 2004 by the Texas Department of State Health Services (formerly Texas Department of Health) in cooperation with Blue Cross and Blue Shield of Texas, the Caring for Children Foundation of Texas, H-E-B (Here Everything's Better) grocery stores, Texas Medical Association, Texas Hospital Association and the American Heart Association of Texas. The goal of the program is to raise awareness of the long-term health risks associated with obesity in adults and children, and to inspire small lifestyle changes that can lead Texans to live healthier lives through exercise and better food choices.

The 2003 Strategic Plan on the Prevention of Obesity in Texas is the basis for the *Building Healthy Families Initiative.* Implementation of this program takes into account the demographic diversity among Texans and the urgency of making overweight and obesity awareness and prevention a part of daily life.

Discussion

Childcare programs can be an effective portal for interventions related to children and eating if the interventions are built upon a mentoring model as described in the previous section of this chapter. However, the content of the mentoring must be focused specifically on children's eating behaviors.

With mentoring, caregivers are shown that they have a unique opportunity to provide nutrition education to children on a continuing basis, rather than through a week-long nutrition unit once or twice during the year. Ideally nutrition and physical activity should be part of the ongoing childcare curriculum.

Nutrition education during the early childhood years is especially important because it is during this period that lifetime eating habits are formed. The quality of nutrition for children 2 to 5 years of age is especially important because it affects their growth and development. Childcare programs need to provide healthy foods that meet recommended dietary guidelines — and offer only those foods to children. Children do not automatically make healthy decisions about food. Without nutrition education and guidance, they tend to choose foods that are high in sodium, salt, sugar and fat, or those foods that are familiar to them. The goal of nutrition education in childcare is to encourage children to make wise choices about the foods they eat.

Childcare providers should be aware that large portion sizes are a major contributing factor in overweight and obesity at all age levels. Providers should serve age-adjusted recommended portions.

Childcare programs should not encourage, force or bribe children to eat more than they actually need. The goal should be for children to learn to self-regulate their food intake — and to realize when they are full and stop eating when satiated.

Caregivers can teach children to recognize the link between nutrition and physical well-being. Children need to be given basic information on the nutrients in foods and their effect on physical growth and development.

Recommendations for caregivers on helping children learn to eat healthy foods in a healthy way include the following:

- Serve children age-appropriate amounts and offer seconds only if the child asks for more.
- Encourage children to eat slowly. Involving children in conversation about foods and eating preferences during snacks and mealtime helps to slow their intake rate and provides an opportunity to discuss nutrition and foods on a daily basis.
- Serve meals and snacks at specific times and remove food when mealtime is over. Some children are naturally slow eaters and may need a few extra minutes to finish the meal.
- Eating should not become a stand-off between caregiver and child. If a child chooses not to eat, then remove the food and tell the child it is time to move on to the next activity. Explain that the child will have another chance to eat at the next snack or mealtime.
- Eating is a behavior that is strongly influenced by the social environment. The eating behavior of other children can serve as a role model and a positive social pressure for influencing a child's food preferences. Seating a child who refuses to eat corn with other children who enjoy eating corn will likely increase the child's willingness to eat corn.
- Caregivers should model what they teach. Do not have coffee, a donut or a can of soda in the room if you expect children to eat healthy food at regular times.

Summary and Conclusions

This chapter discussed using childcare programs as a portal for interventions to change children's eating behaviors, focusing specifically on mentoring of providers as an intervention model. I provided details on an empirical study of mentoring, a randomized clinical trial of mentoring in Pennsylvania childcare programs.

The mentoring model is an approach that all 50 states can use as all have training systems that are funded through the Federal Child Care Development Fund. Unfortunately, the predominant training approach in childcare programs remains traditional workshops that have been demonstrated to be ineffective in training interventions. Although mentoring does cost more to deliver, the effectiveness of this approach offsets its expense. A mentoring approach that focuses on children's eating behaviors during the hours they spend in childcare can be a very effective intervention strategy for producing positive changes in these specific behaviors.

References

1. Breunig R, Bellm A. *Early Childhood Mentoring Programs: A Survey of Community Initiatives.* Washington, DC: Center for the Child Care Workforce; 1996.
2. Fenichel I. *Learning Through Supervision and Mentorship.* Washington, DC: Zero to Three: National Center for Infants, Toddlers and Families; 1992.
3. Fiene R. Improving child care quality through an infant caregiver mentoring project. *Child and Youth Care Forum.* 2002;31:75-83.
4. Iutcovich J, Fiene R, Johnson J, Koppel R, Langan F. *Investing in Our Children's Future.* Erie, Pa: Keystone University Research Corp; 1997.
5. Johnson J. *Child Care Training and Developmentally Appropriate Beliefs and Practices of Child Care Employees in Pennsylvania.* Harrisburg, Pa: Center for Schools and Communities; 1994.
6. Fiene R, Greenberg M, Bergsten M, Carl B, Fegley C, Gibbons L. *The Pennsylvania Early Childhood Quality Settings Study.* Harrisburg, Pa: Governor's Task Force on Early Care and Education; 2002.
7. Hresko W, Miguel S, Sherbenou R. Burton S. *Developmental Observation Checklist System (DOCS).* Austin, Texas: Pro-ed Publishing; 1994.
8. North Carolina Cooperative Extension. Color Me Healthy. 2003. Available at: http://www.ces.ncsu.edu/wake/fee/nutrition/colorhealthy.htm. Accessed December 21, 2006.
9. New York State Department of Health. Eat Well Play Hard. 2005. Available at: http://www.health.state.ny.us/prevention/nutrition/resources/ewph.htm. Accessed December 21, 2006.
10. Texas Department of State Heakth Services. Building Healthy Families Initiatives. 2004. Available at: http://www.dshs.state.tx.us/dshstoday/obesity.shtm. Acccessed December 21, 2006.

Section 4
Summary

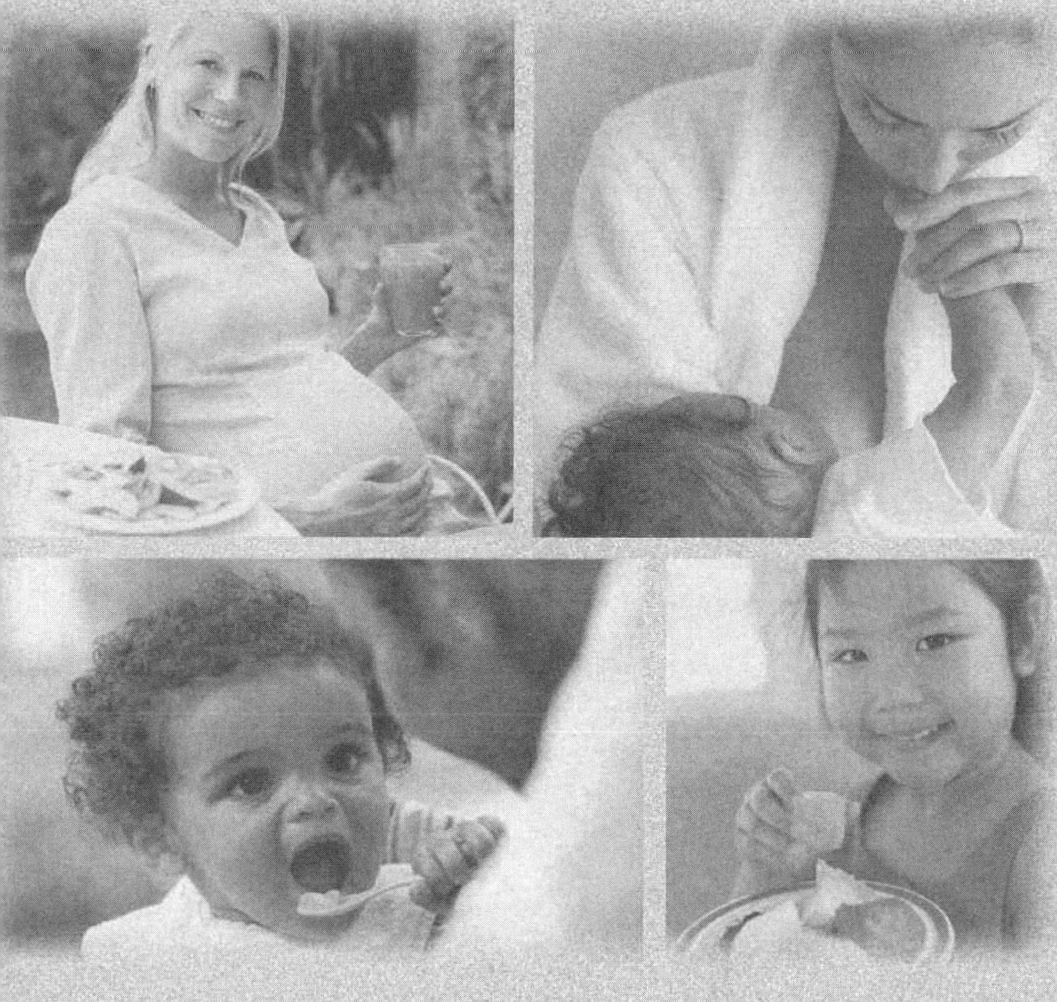

Eating Behaviors of the Young Child Practices and Interventions

William Dietz, MD, PhD

The findings and conclusions in this report are those of the author and do not necessarily represent the views of the Centers for Disease Control and Prevention.

The chapters included in this volume address a variety of factors that influence feeding of infants and young children that may contribute to later obesity and other chronic diseases. In utero exposure to the maternal diet, breastfeeding and the exposure to the maternal diet that occurs through breast milk, sensitivity to infant cues, television viewing and parental modeling all appear to have an impact on infant food preferences. Furthermore, parents' interpretations of infants' satiety cues may influence both infants' and children's abilities to regulate their intake. In addition, although few systematic studies have been done, qualitative data suggest that there are marked cultural differences in parental willingness to concede food choices to children when children refuse the foods that are offered. All of these factors are likely to play a role in the types of foods that infants consume and the quality of their diet, and ultimately may determine how susceptible they are to excessive weight gain.

Helping Parents Shape Children's Diets

While there was consensus among the authors on the importance of all these factors in shaping the quality of children's diets and ultimately contributing to their overall health, there are few clinical interventions that positively address feeding practices.

What is currently available to guide parents in feeding their children? The American Academy of Pediatrics (AAP) and the American Dietetic Association, with the support of the Food Marketing Institute, jointly developed several brochures on infant feeding problems some 15 years ago. These pamphlets were based on clinical judgment and experience rather than qualitative research with diverse populations — and they were never pretested with parents. Nonetheless, these pamphlets are still available from the AAP and are among their more popular parent brochures. Their effectiveness in changing parental behavior remains uncertain.

Because so few educational materials on child feeding exist, and because parenting practices appear to be increasingly important determinants of diet, physical activity levels and television viewing habits in young children, the AAP and the Johnson & Johnson Pediatric Institute, L.L.C. (JJPI) agreed to use the ideas and directions that grew out of a Pediatric Round Table on Eating Behaviors of the Young Child to develop new, culturally appropriate materials for parents. These materials will be based on strategies and gaps identified during the conference, as well as a subsequent survey of parents of young children. Every effort will be made to assure that they are culturally appropriate, including pretesting them with parents from various population groups prior to final development and distribution.

The parenting practices most relevant to the early prevention of overweight are likely those that affect decisions about feeding (breastfeeding, introducing solid foods and limiting the intake of sugar-sweetened beverages) and other lifestyle decisions (encouraging physical activity and limiting television viewing). Practices that simultaneously target several of these areas may be particularly helpful. For example, reductions in television viewing may affect both dietary intake and activity levels. In addition, efforts to reinforce the intake of foods that are traditional to a culture might be enhanced by emphasizing to parents that an infant's cultural heritage begins with exposure to the flavors of those traditional foods in the maternal diet that are transmitted to the infant through the amniotic fluid or breast milk. An alternative message is that infants may be more likely to accept traditional foods later on if they are breastfed as infants, because the flavors of the maternal diet are transmitted to the infant through breast milk.

The family meal is also a potentially productive target for positively influencing parental feeding practices. A recent Kaiser Family Foundation report on children and television[1] and qualitative research supported by the Centers for Disease Control and Prevention[2] indicate that more than 50% of families watch television while eating. Furthermore, the relationship between television time and the risk of childhood overweight is widely recognized. Finally, children in families that have family meals together have healthier diets and lower incidence of obesity than do children from families that do not have family meals.[3,4] Because families value family time, promotion of family meals without television may accomplish several goals: increase family bonding, improve diet quality, and reduce the risk of excess weight gain because of improved diet quality and reduced television time. Whether the promotion of family meals achieves any of these posited outcomes remains uncertain, but promotion of family meals clearly offers a promising approach for practice and further research.

Another critical area that has an effect on the risk of child overweight relates to parental feeding practices. For example, portion size appears to influence food intake in normal weight and overweight males and females across age groups. Observational and clinical experiences suggest that parents often serve children inappropriately large portions and then become concerned when children do not consume all the food that is offered. Conflicts between parents and children about whether they have had enough to eat, the consumption of fruits and vegetables and/or the use of dessert to promote greater food consumption also are promising targets for intervention.

One strategy that addresses these conflicts is to promote the division of responsibility between parents and children around food intake.[5,6] The division of responsibility assigns to parents the responsibility for the kind of food that is offered and to children the decision of whether or not to consume the food that is offered and what quantity they should consume. Several elements are key to the effective implementation of this strategy. If a child decides not to eat what is offered, it is not up to the parent to offer an alternative. Parents often are concerned that if their children do not eat what is offered, they will be hungry. Although that is true, hunger that is the logical consequence of food refusal makes it much more likely that the child will consume the refused food when it is offered again. The appropriate parental response is to put the food aside and tell the child that if he or she becomes hungry later, the food will be available for them then. If parents are consistent in the application of the division of responsibility with the child, they can minimize conflicts.

There are several important barriers to the implementation of these positive feeding strategies:

- Many parents are not aware of appropriate portion sizes for infants and toddlers, do not appreciate the substantial day-to-day variability in intake or food preferences, or are not persistent in the introduction of new foods because they may not understand that multiple offerings of new foods are essential before they are accepted.
- Parents also may misinterpret infant facial expressions in response to new foods as distaste for new foods, misinterpret infant cues related to satiety, or are not convinced that the child can adequately regulate satiation.

How Can Healthcare Providers Better Counsel Parents on Feeding Issues?

One of the first strategies is to improve the abilities of pediatric healthcare providers to counsel parents. The two products that grew out of the Pediatric Round Table conference on children and feeding begin that process. As indicated above, the educational material for parents that is being developed will complement and expand upon the AAP brochure developed 15 years ago. The strengths of the new material include the increased understanding of infant feeding practices presented at the conference, as well as information related to parental needs gathered from parents in a survey designed as part of the process, and from pretesting the brochure with parents for clarity and relevance. In addition, the chapters of this book provide pediatric practitioners with latest knowledge from experts in early childhood nutrition and feeding, activity and television viewing.

Primary care offers one important setting to reach parents, counsel them and help them change behaviors that predispose children to excessive weight gain. Although the products of this conference fill an important gap in education, education alone may not be sufficient to change the behavior of either parents or providers. Motivational interviewing, a method of proven effectiveness in the treatment of addictive behaviors, has been successfully pilot tested as a tool to change parenting around nutrition and food intake.[7] However, the efficacy of motivational interviewing in changing behaviors around nutrition, physical activity and/or television viewing has not yet been demonstrated. Even if motivational interviewing proves efficacious, its dissemination, uptake and effective application by primary care providers remains uncertain. Despite these challenges, parental counseling by primary care providers remains an important option to improve parenting practices around feeding, physical activity and television viewing.

Public Health Approaches to Preventing Child Obesity

Public health approaches to improve parenting practices with young children around nutrition, physical activity and television viewing have received even less attention. Another dimension of the potential effects of parenting was suggested by a recent paper that linked general parenting style to the likelihood of overweight in children in a large group of subjects.[8] Parenting styles were classified based on maternal sensitivity to children's needs and maternal expectations for their child's self-control. Parenting styles were described as authoritarian, when strict disciplinary practices were employed; authoritative, when clear rules were present but the child's opinions were respected; permissive, when parenting was indulgent without discipline; or neglectful, when families were emotionally uninvolved. The risk of overweight was greatest among children in families with authoritarian parenting styles, followed by children exposed to permissive or neglectful parenting. The lowest prevalence of overweight occurred among children whose parents had an authoritative style. How these parenting styles translate to practices related to feeding, physical activity and television viewing remains a subject for further research. Furthermore, how the impact of parenting style varies with ethnicity, whether these styles can be changed through counseling provided in primary care settings — and whether these changes would reduce the risk of overweight — has not yet been studied.

Authoritarian, permissive and neglectful parenting styles may be associated with other adverse health outcomes for children. One program designed to improve parenting is an approach known as the "Triple P" or the Positive Parenting Practices program. This program, developed in Australia, was designed to improve parenting practices. The program consists of a flexible approach that enables various levels of intervention and intensity, depending on the severity of the problem.[9,10] This approach is only beginning to be applied to parenting around diet[11] but is a method that potentially has a wider reach than primary care approaches.

Onset of overweight in early childhood may contribute disproportionately to the risk of severe overweight in adulthood. Excessive food intake, inactivity and television viewing predispose children to excessive weight gain. As was discussed at the Pediatric Round Table, and is further elaborated on in these chapters, parenting practices are major determinants of food intake, food quality and television viewing. Physical activity was not extensively addressed at this conference, but at least as many factors are likely to affect energy expenditure as affect energy intake. Efforts to improve parenting practices related to food choices and activity may, therefore, offer opportunities to prevent the early onset of overweight. Unfortunately, few settings provide opportunities to discuss or change parenting practices. We thank JJPI for sponsorship of this ground breaking meeting. The AAP is to be congratulated for their willingness to use the products from it to try to achieve changes in parental feeding practices. At the very least, this systematic approach to the development of new materials for parents moves these efforts forward. Furthermore, we hope that the Round Table and its proceedings will inspire both attendees and the readers of this book to develop new and improved strategies to help parents make more appropriate food and activity choices for their children.

References

1. Rideout V, Hamel E. *The Media Family: Electronic Media in the Lives of Infants, Toddlers, Preschoolers, and Their Parents.* Menlo Park, Calif: Kaiser Family; 2005.
2. Jordan AB, Hersey JC, McDivitt JA, Heitzler CD. Reducing children's television-viewing time: a qualitative study of parents and their children. *Pediatrics.* 2006;118:1303-1310.
3. Taveras EM, Rifas-Shiman SL, Berkey CS, et al. Family dinner and adolescent overweight. *Obesity Research.* 2005;13:900-906.
4. Gillman MW, Rifas-Shiman SL, Camargo CA Jr, Field AE, Berkey CS, Colditz GA. Family dinner and diet quality among older children and adolescents. *Archives of Family Medicine.* 2000;9:235-240.
5. Satter E. *How to Get Your Kid to Eat...But Not Too Much.* Palo Alto, Calif: Bull Publishing Company; 1987.
6. Dietz WH, Stern L. *Guide to Your Child's Nutrition.* New York, NY: Villard; 1999.
7. Schwartz RP, Hamre R, Dietz WH, et al. Office-based motivational interviewing to prevent childhood obesity: a feasibility study. *Pediatrics.* In press.
8. Rhee KE, Lumeng JC, Appugliese DP, Kaciroti N, Bradley RH. Parenting styles and overweight in first grade. *Pediatrics.* 2006;117:2047-2054.
9. Sanders MR. Triple P – Positive Parenting Program: a population approach to promoting competent parenting. *Australian e-Journal for the Advancement of Mental Health* [serial online]. 2003;2(3):2. Available at: http://www.auseinet.com/journal/vol2iss3/sanders.pdf. Accessed January 23, 2007.

10. Sanders MR, Markie-Dadds C, Turner KMT. Theoretical, scientific and clinical foundations of the Triple P – Positive Parenting Program: a population approach to the promotion of parenting competence. Parenting Research and Practice Monograph No. 1. Available at: http://www5.triplep.net/. Accessed January 23, 2007.
11. Golley RK, Magarey AM, Baur LA, Steinbeck, KS, Daniels LA. Twelve-month effectiveness of a parent-led, family-focused weight management program for pre-pubertal children: a randomized controlled trial. *Pediatrics.* In press.